QUALITATIVE RESEAR
FOR OCCUPATIONAL
PHYSICAL THERAPIS
A PRACTICAL GUIDE

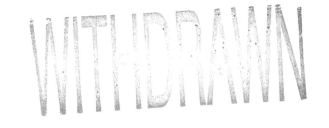

QUALITATIVE RESEARCH FOR OCCUPATIONAL AND PHYSICAL THERAPISTS: A PRACTICAL GUIDE

Christine Carpenter Ph.D., MA, BA, DipPT

Reader in Physiotherapy, Faculty of Health and Life Sciences, Coventry University, Coventry, UK

Melinda Suto Ph.D., MA, BS

Assistant Professor, Department of Occupational Sciences and Occupational Therapy, University of British Columbia, Vancouver, Canada

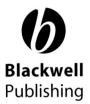

Blackwell
Publishing

Blackwell Publishing editorial offices:

Blackwell Publishing Ltd, 9600 Garsington Road, Oxford OX4 2DQ, UK
   Tel: +44 (0)1865 776868
Blackwell Publishing Professional, 2121 State Avenue, Ames, Iowa 50014-8300, USA
   Tel: +1 515 292 0140
Blackwell Publishing Asia Pty Ltd, 550 Swanston Street, Carlton, Victoria 3053, Australia
   Tel: +61 (0)3 8359 1011

First published 2008 by Blackwell Publishing Ltd

ISBN-13: 978-1-4051-4435-3

Library of Congress Cataloging-in-Publication Data

Carpenter, Christine, DipPT.
   Qualitative research for occupational and physical therapy : a practical guide / Christine
Carpenter, Melinda Suto.
      p. ; cm.
   Includes bibliographical references and index.
   ISBN-13: 978-1-4051-4435-3 (pbk. : alk. paper)
   1. Occupational therapy—Research—Methodology.   2. Physical therapy—
Research—Methodology.   3. Qualitative research.   I. Suto, Melinda.   II. Title.
   [DNLM: 1. Occupational Therapy.   2. Physical Therapy (Specialty)   3. Data Collection.
4. Qualitative Research.   5. Research Design.   WB 460 C295q 2008]
   RM735.42.C37 2008
   615.8′515072—dc22

                                                                                  2007044468

A catalogue record for this title is available from the British Library

Set in 10/12.5pt Sabon by Graphicraft Limited, Hong Kong
Printed and bound in Singapore by COS Printers Pte Ltd

The publisher's policy is to use permanent paper from mills that operate a sustainable forestry
policy, and which has been manufactured from pulp processed using acid-free and elementary
chlorine-free practices. Furthermore, the publisher ensures that the text paper and cover board
used have met acceptable environmental accreditation standards.

For further information on Blackwell Publishing, visit our website:
www.blackwellpublishing.com

CONTENTS

AUTHOR INFORMATION

Chris Carpenter was educated as a physical therapist in Liverpool, England, and attained her graduate degrees in Educational Studies at the University of British Columbia (UBC), Canada. Before joining the School of Rehabilitation Sciences at UBC she worked for over 20 years in rehabilitation settings primarily with individuals who had sustained spinal cord injury. In 2004 she relocated to the United Kingdom and is currently a Reader in Physiotherapy in the Faculty of Health and Life Sciences, Coventry University. She has extensive experience teaching at both graduate and undergraduate levels (including qualitative research methodologies and methods) and has received several university teaching awards. Dr Carpenter is also involved in providing supervision for research projects for undergraduate and graduate students in the United Kingdom, Canada and the United States of America. Her current research initiatives focus on the long-term experience and quality of life issues following spinal cord injury, dilemmas of professional practice in rehabilitation settings and interdisciplinary education. She is an editor and author with Karen Hammell of *Using Qualitative Research: A Practical Introduction for Occupational and Physical Therapists* (2000) and of *Qualitative Research in Evidence-based Rehabilitation* (2004).

Melinda Suto was educated in California, and attained a bachelor's degree at San Jose State University, a master's degree at the University of Southern California, and a Ph.D. in Educational Studies at the University of British Columbia (UBC), Canada. Before joining the Department of Occupational Science and Occupational Therapy at UBC, she worked primarily with clients experiencing mental health problems and now teaches qualitative research methodologies and methods to graduate students. Presently she is conducting research focused on how everyday occupations, such as leisure activities, work performance, and friendships, are influenced by the psychosocial aspects of bipolar disorder. Her previous research explored leisure meanings created by women who immigrated to Canada and their participation in leisure activities. Other interests cover a broad range of community mental health issues such as stigma, conceptual development in occupational science and occupational therapy, and client-practitioner communication such as the informed shared decision-making process. She has contributed chapters to books co-edited by Karen Hammell and Chris Carpenter.

PREFACE

Evidence-based practice has emerged as one of the most influential concepts in health care in the past decade but 'best' evidence continues to be defined as being derived from 'scientific' quantitative research approaches. Compelling arguments are being made, particularly in health care and education, to broaden the scope of evidence-based practice, and there is a move to recognize the contribution that qualitative research approaches can make to theory building, directing and evaluating service and program provision, and developing and implementing relevant and effective interventions. In addition, practitioners working with rehabilitation clients who have an injury or chronic condition have identified a lack of congruence between standardized outcome measures and effectiveness research with the philosophy of client-centered practice and the experiences of clients in their real contexts and over their lifespan.

It is becoming clear that rigorous qualitative research can effectively address contemporary concerns about accountability and the provision of best practice. Qualitative research is especially appropriate as a means of investigating the central and complex issues of rehabilitation: quality of life, aging, management of impairment and the experience of chronic illness in the long term, client-directed care and self-management, effective patient education and interdisciplinary team functioning. These are issues which form a major component of rehabilitation practice, but which have been long neglected in research owing to their incompatibility with traditional forms of scientific inquiry.

Despite an exponential growth of interest in qualitative research approaches in health care there continues to be a scarcity of books that address these methodologies from the perspective of occupational therapists and physical therapists with specific reference to the provision of rehabilitation services in institutional and community settings. To date, rehabilitation practitioners have been required to access resources primarily from sociology, anthropology and education, and in health from the nursing literature.

As instructors in occupational therapy and physical therapy education programs, we teach qualitative research methodology and methods within academic cultures that have traditionally 'privileged' quantitative research in terms of both curriculum content and the resources supporting it. It was the need to clearly articulate the fundamentals of qualitative research design and implementation in relation to occupational therapy and physical therapy practice that motivated us to write this book. The aim of *Qualitative Research for Occupational and Physical Therapists: A Practical Guide* is to facilitate the knowledge and skills required to address the practicalities of conducting and evaluating qualitative research with, and for the benefit of, clients using rehabilitation services. This book encourages readers to share our enthusiasm for these research approaches and the substantial contribution rigorous qualitative research can make to practice. In this book we will critically explore the theoretical context of rehabilitation practice and the qualitative approaches relevant to health care research, and assist the reader to make the informed methodological and method choices needed to address research questions, ensure the trustworthiness of the study, and to conduct research in an ethical manner.

The book is organized in the form of ten chapters that together present, in a logical fashion, the intellectual and practical process that researchers engage in when developing and implementing a qualitative research study. Current examples of qualitative research studies in occupational therapy and physical therapy will be used to illustrate core concepts and the contribution qualitative research can make to rehabilitation practice.

Chapter 1 introduces and defines qualitative research, discusses the importance of theory to the research endeavor and establishes the theoretical context of rehabilitation and the contribution qualitative research can make to client-centered and evidence-based practice.

Chapter 2 discusses the philosophical systems that form the foundation of qualitative research and explores the assumptions that characterize qualitative research and its role in connecting theory to practice.

Chapter 3 outlines the process of planning a qualitative research project and the decisions that need to be made in order to develop an original and relevant, yet realistic, research topic. Each of the components outlined in this chapter are discussed in more detail in subsequent chapters.

Chapter 4 discusses the importance of examining and matching the theoretical traditions or methodological approaches to qualitative inquiry, for example phenomenology, to the substantive issue being investigated.

Chapter 5 discusses the practicalities of involving participants in qualitative research and obtaining ethical approval and reviews a number of methods of data collection.

Chapter 6 discusses the nature and different forms of qualitative data and effective ways of organizing and managing it.

Chapter 7 discusses the reflexive and interpretive nature of the qualitative data analysis process and describes a foundational thematic approach to analysis.

Chapter 8 describes the process through which the researcher moves from data collection and analysis to disseminating the findings, with a particular emphasis on the issues of representation and accountability.

Chapter 9 explores the judicious use of evaluative criteria and strategies designed to ensure and evaluate the trustworthiness and credibility of qualitative research.

Chapter 10 discusses future developments in qualitative research related to the participant–researcher relationship characteristic of qualitative research, the increasing use of mixed methods research approaches, meta-synthesis of qualitative research findings, and use of the Internet and email by qualitative researchers.

Christine Carpenter
Coventry, United Kingdom, 2007

Melinda Suto
Vancouver, Canada, 2007

ACKNOWLEDGMENTS

We would like to acknowledge the support and encouragement we received from Karen Hammell and Clare Taylor. Dr Hammell collaborated in developing the initial proposal for this book and has graciously shared her ideas and resources with us. Dr Taylor is an innovative teacher of qualitative research and this book has benefited from her experience and generous contribution of teaching materials.

Chapter 1

QUALITATIVE RESEARCH IN THE REHABILITATION CONTEXT

Introduction: what is qualitative research?

The question 'What is qualitative research?' is frequently asked by occupational therapists and physical therapists,[1] or students exploring, for the first time, the possibility of developing a research idea or question and designing a study to address it effectively. The response to the question is, however, a complicated one. This complexity can be traced to a number of sources, such as the trans-disciplinary nature of qualitative inquiry, the historical contest between the proponents of quantitative and qualitative research approaches, the emergence of qualitative research in health care, and the challenge of evidence-based practice. In our experience, this complexity and the need to grapple with it elicits different reactions from rehabilitation practitioners and students. For some, the theoretical foundations and assumptions of qualitative research approaches appear congruent with their practice philosophy and questions. For others, qualitative inquiry represents a very different "worldview",[2] one that is unsettling and difficult to comprehend as it challenges the dominant traditional assumptions about the nature and purpose of research, and requires us to reflect critically on the professional and theoretical assumptions influencing rehabilitation practice. In this chapter, we will establish a broad definition of qualitative research and discuss the theoretical context within which rehabilitation practice takes place. Increasingly, qualitative research studies are being reported in the occupational therapy and physical therapy literature, and it is our intention to take advantage of these resources as examples throughout this book.

Defining qualitative research

Qualitative research is historically associated with anthropology, sociology, education and psychology; it is a field of inquiry separate and distinct from survey

---

[1] Physical therapy is the term used in the United States and physiotherapy is most commonly used outside North America. The terms can be considered synonymous. For consistency, physical therapy will be used in this book.

[2] Double quotation marks will be used throughout this book to indicate contentious terms that we consider need to be used critically.

and other forms of quantitative research. As a result, it cuts across disciplines, subject matters and practice areas. Qualitative research is an umbrella term for the concepts, assumptions and methods shared by a complex and interconnected family of research traditions and it has meant different things at different points in its history.

Throughout the nineteenth century and until World War II, qualitative researchers, particularly in sociology and anthropology, were concerned with producing valid, reliable and objective knowledge, reflective of the positivist paradigm about strange and foreign worlds (for example Malinowski, 1922). As a result, qualitative research in many, if not all its forms (observation, participation, interviewing, ethnography) came to be associated with the classification of indigenous people and the worst excesses of colonization (Denzin & Lincoln, 2005). During the period from the post-war years to the late 1970s many efforts were made to develop interpretive approaches, such as feminism, phenomenology and critical theory, and to formalize qualitative methods in an attempt to justify the rigor of qualitative approaches to research. Qualitative research began to be adopted in health care, primarily by medical sociology (for example Becker *et al.*, 1961) and nursing (for example Field & Morse, 1985) during this period. There was an emphasis on the standardization of data collection methods, such as the development of participant observation forms, and a more quantitative approach to data analysis through the use of 'quasi-statistics', such as word or code frequencies. Such structured approaches to data analysis were most graphically illustrated in Glaser & Strauss' (1967) work *The Discovery of Grounded Theory*, and later two books by Geertz, *The Interpretation of Cultures* (1973) and *Local Knowledge* (1983), were particularly influential. During the 1980s, there was a general move away from the influence of the positivist discourse and in the 1990s, qualitative researchers, particularly in health care, experienced what might be called an identity crisis. New models of "truth", method and representation were sought and issues of objectivity, reliability, validity and generalizability once again became problematic (Denzin & Lincoln, 2005). During this period, qualitative research seemed to have arrived in the research mainstream, with increasing discussion and recognition occurring in medical and other health profession journals and the publication of new journals such as *Qualitative Health Research*.

In the twenty-first century, the field of qualitative research continues to be a dynamic one, and the use of evaluative criteria in judging the quality, trustworthiness and credibility of qualitative research studies remains controversial and the topic of much debate by qualitative research theorists. A number of influential authors (Denzin & Lincoln, 2005; Miller & Crabtree, 2005) have articulated new challenges for qualitative researchers related to the concept of evidence-based practice in medicine and, in the United States, to the scientifically based research movement or "Bush science". This movement places experimental quantitative research first among scientific methods in policy statements and relegates qualitative approaches to an auxiliary role (Bloch, 2004; Howe, 2004). This, according to Denzin & Lincoln (2005), 'endorses a narrow view of science' (p. 9) and 'has created a hostile environment for qualitative research' (p. 8). Despite these recent challenging developments, Miller & Crabtree (2005) remain convinced that qualitative clinical research is now widely accepted in health care, including medicine. Over the past decade there has been growing theoretical discussion and debate about the congruence of qualitative research with occupational therapy practice (for example Hammell, 2001; Bailey & Jackson, 2003; Ballinger, 2004). The physical therapy profession has been slower to recognize the potential contribution of qualitative research to our understanding of practice (Robertson, 1994; Bithell, 2000) and critical debate in the physical therapy literature remains more limited (for example Shepard *et al.*, 1993; Carpenter, 1997; Johnson & Waterfield, 2004).

All of which brings us back to the thorny problem of defining qualitative research! As Denzin & Lincoln (2005) assert, 'any definition of qualitative research must work within this complex historical [context]' (p. 3). These authors suggest the following generic definition:

> Qualitative research is a situated activity that locates the observer in the world. It consists of a set of interpretive, material practices that make the world [the taken for granted in everyday life] visible [to others]. Qualitative research involves the studied use and collection of a variety of empirical information using a diversity of methods, for example case study, personal narrative, artifacts, cultural texts, interviews, observations, and visual records that describe routine and problematic moments in individuals' lives with the aim of developing a better understanding of the subject or phenomenon. Qualitative research privileges no single methodological practice over another and has no theory or paradigm that is distinctly its own (pp. 5–6).

This definition suggests an interpretive, naturalistic research approach that uses multiple sources of information and is grounded in a number of philosophical assumptions. Creswell's (1998) definition conveys similar ideas but focuses more on the elements that characterize qualitative research approaches:

> Qualitative research is an inquiry process of understanding based on distinct methodological traditions of inquiry that explore a social or human problem. The researcher builds a complex, holistic picture, analyzes words, reports detailed views of informants, and conducts the study in the natural setting (p. 15).

In health care, discussions of qualitative research have largely focused on comparing and contrasting it with assumptions, techniques and strategies developed for quantitative research (Bogdan & Biklen, 1998; Hammell *et al.*, 2000). However, as Creswell (1998) firmly states, 'qualitative inquiry represents a legitimate mode of social and human science exploration without apology or comparisons to quantitative research' (p. 9).

While a certain amount of comparison is unavoidable, in this book we have attempted to concentrate on what qualitative research *is* rather than presenting what it *is not* and on considering the differences among approaches to qualitative research. There is no "best" approach to research; rather it depends on what is being studied and on the nature of the research question. In a qualitative study, the research question often starts with *how* or *what*, and aims to describe or explore what is going on. This is in contrast to quantitative questions that ask *why*, and aim to make comparisons between groups or explain cause and effect relationships between variables (Creswell, 1998). According to Miller & Crabtree (2005) the guiding premise of clinical research is that 'the questions emerging from the embodied, embedded, and mindfully lived clinical experience frame conversations and determine research design [decisions]' (p. 609). The word 'research' is derived from the Middle French verb *recercher*, meaning 'to go about seeking' and is variously defined in the Merriam-Webster Online Dictionary (2006) as:

- The collection of information about a particular topic or phenomenon
- Careful or diligent search for explanation or information
- Studious inquiry or examination: especially the investigation or experimentation aimed at the discovery and interpretation of facts, revision of accepted theories or laws in the light of new facts, or the practical application and evaluation of such new or revised theories or laws
- To search or investigate exhaustively

Conducting research, then, has multiple aims and these diverse definitions support the argument that in the rapidly changing and increasingly accountable world of health care no one research approach can be privileged over others. Multiple research approaches are needed if the ongoing generation of new knowledge, and search for evidence about the effectiveness of professional practice, is to be supported. Thus, it is imperative that practitioners develop an in-depth knowledge of different research approaches in order to be critical consumers of research.

The field of qualitative research, like any specialty area, has cultivated a language and terminology that practitioners and students may initially find off-putting and daunting and which, almost assuredly, excludes health care clients from the research dialogue. We learn the distinct languages and professional jargon of occupational therapy and physical therapy as part of the enculturation process to the professions. Similarly, learning the language of qualitative research facilitates our in-depth understanding of the research process and enables us to explain and share our new understanding with clients and research participants. It is our intention in this book to facilitate this learning process by making the qualitative research terms and concepts accessible to the reader.

Issues of theory in qualitative research

The aim of this book is to facilitate the knowledge and skills occupational therapists and physical therapists need in order to address the practicalities of conducting and evaluating qualitative research with, and for the benefit of, clients using rehabilitation services. However, the research endeavor is not an atheoretical one and before addressing the practicalities of research, we need to explore the different theoretical perspectives influencing rehabilitation practice. Hammell (2006) suggests that rehabilitation practitioners rarely question 'the taken-for-granted nature of traditional knowledge and assumptions within the rehabilitation, health and community care industries' or 'contest, critique or challenge the way in which disability [physical and psychological] is understood and managed' (p. ix). The central issue of theory in qualitative research can be troubling, particularly for those of us primarily educated in the positivist paradigm and quantitative method (Dyck, 2000), where researcher "objectivity" is paramount. Qualitative research, in contrast, is based on the premise that researchers do not enter the research process as a "blank page". Even if researchers are unaware of their theoretical orientation, or how these issues may influence the proposed study, their choice of research topic and design is necessarily framed by a perspective laden with ideas and concepts arising from a particular professional body of knowledge, and experience in a specific field of practice, as well as personal experiences (Dyck, 2000). Two examples may help to elucidate what we mean by influence. In exploring the lived experience of disability with participants who had sustained traumatic spinal cord injuries, Carpenter (1994) came to recognize for the first time in a long career as a physical therapist in rehabilitation, how dominant disability theories, in particular stages of adjustment and the personal tragedy model of disability (Swain & French, 2000), had influenced her practice and attitudes towards the value systems of clients in rehabilitation that gave rise to their personal goals and aspirations. Dyck (2000), an occupational therapist, discusses how ideas from social theory, particularly those developed in feminist scholarship, helped her in analyzing women's workplace experiences following a diagnosis of multiple sclerosis.

According to Denzin & Lincoln (2005) all qualitative researchers are philosophers, in the sense that they are guided by highly abstract beliefs and feelings about the nature of human beings, reality and knowledge. This comprises a conceptual framework that shapes how we view the world and how it should be understood and studied. Such beliefs may be taken for granted, invisible, or merely assumed, whereas others may be revealed as highly problematic and controversial. Therefore, from a qualitative research perspective, all research is interpretive and not a neutral or objective undertaking. We will address these important issues in more detail later in the book in relation to the purpose of research, the dissemination of research findings and the role of the researcher in the process.

The professional context

The values, beliefs and principles of a discipline have a major influence on its identity and development, and are known collectively as its philosophy (Baum & Christiansen, 1997). A profession's philosophy focuses on providing the framework for asking both ontological and epistemological questions about the central values, assumptions, concepts and actions that are the foundation of practice. Examples of ontological questions are, 'What is the nature of reality?' Alternatively,

'What does it mean to be human?' *Ontology*[3] is the study of being or existence, of conceptions of reality. It is from these ontological concerns that epistemological questions arise. *Epistemology* is concerned with theories of knowledge, beliefs about the nature of knowledge, the process by which knowledge is acquired and the reliability of claims to knowledge (Hammell, 2006). A professional philosophy – including such concepts as respect for autonomy and quality of life – is instilled in the process of acquiring an identity as a nurse, occupational therapist, physical therapist or physician. However, the philosophical and historical roots that shape practice are articulated in varying degrees by different professions. For example, according to some authors in physical therapy (Roskell *et al.*, 1998; Richardson, 1999), the values and priorities held by the physical therapy profession today are rarely explored in the literature or taught in the academic programs. The acquisition of knowledge, skills, values, roles and attitudes associated with the practice of a particular profession occurs through a process of professional socialization. This process begins during the period of formal education and continues through interaction with others in a variety of clinical settings. It represents the development of a unique voice and professional view of the world based on, to a greater or lesser degree, shared assumptions.

According to Hammell (2006), among rehabilitation professionals, these shared *assumptions* 'concern the nature of their work (apolitical, relevant and useful), the nature of their goals (increasing function, performance and independence to enhance quality of life) and the caliber of their relationships with . . . patients and clients (benevolent, client-centered and helpful)' (p. 3). These assumptions represent a set of taken-for-granted statements that organized together form a theory of rehabilitation practice. Such a *theory* can be defined as a framework or system of explanatory principles or ideas that describe, explain, predict or prescribe responses, events, situations or relationships within a specific reality. It is, by definition, speculative and, even when unacknowledged or unstated, informs professional practice (Hammell, 2006). What is not clear is whether these theoretical assumptions and beliefs about rehabilitation practice have a supportive evidence base. Concerns have been raised in the nursing and rehabilitation sciences literature (Fealy, 1997; Roskell *et al.*, 1998) about the perceived widening theory–practice gap. In physical therapy, this gap has been attributed to a poorly articulated and understood professional philosophy and a reliance on positivist approaches to scientific inquiry, resulting in a narrow and incomplete body of evidence (De Souza, 1998; Roskell *et al.*, 1998). Two survey studies highlight concerns related to the use of theory and evidence in practice; one study sought to examine the approaches used in stroke rehabilitation by occupational therapists (Walker *et al.*, 2000) and the other focused on physical therapists (Davidson & Waters, 2000). The two most common approaches used by occupational therapists were the functional approach and the Bobath approach. The main indications

---

[3] Terms which are uniquely associated with qualitative research and may be new to the reader will be italicized the first time they are introduced in the book.

for the choice of approach were the age of the patient, progress with other approaches and discharge date. Walker *et al.* (2000) expressed concern that, in the current climate of evidence-based practice, a high number of the survey respondents were unable to describe adequately the theoretical basis for the treatment used. Davidson & Waters (2000) found that there was a great deal of variation in the beliefs held by physical therapists about the treatment of stroke patients even though the Bobath approach was by far the most dominant treatment approach used. These diverse interpretations of how the Bobath approach is applied were unsubstantiated by reference to published evidence.

Findings like these are a concern when we consider that practice (clinical observation and logical speculation) guides theory development, which in turn guides research. Theory provides researchers with a basis for developing lines of inquiry by which practice can be critically investigated and changed. However, some authors (Albrecht & Devlieger, 1999; Johnstone, 2001; Hammell, 2006) argue that the theories of rehabilitation espoused by rehabilitation professionals have been uncritically accepted, are restrictive in nature, and their influence on research is poorly articulated. Traditionally, rehabilitation professionals have privileged their own assumptions, perspectives and knowledge in directing rehabilitation research and services, even though these are frequently unacknowledged and not clearly articulated (Hammell, 2006).

The context of rehabilitation

Corbet (2000) produced a movie about people's experiences of rehabilitation and described a theme common to everyone's story. This theme was 'that early on they'd been told more about what they couldn't do than what they could do' (p. 4). It seemed that rehabilitation practitioners had chosen not only to share their knowledge about physical impairments, for example the ability, or in this case the inability, to walk after a spinal cord injury, but also their beliefs about more general societal roles and capabilities that, in their view, would no longer be possible for the clients, for example having children and becoming employed. Such client experiences graphically illustrate aspects of the dominant theoretical models of disability that continue to influence the delivery of rehabilitation services. A *model* is a conceptual framework that encapsulates, and posits links between, specific knowledge and concepts. Models, according to Finkelstein (2004), act as tools to give us insights into situations that would otherwise be difficult to begin to explain. This section will outline the assumptions of several models of disability and rehabilitation, introduce related key concepts, and briefly examine the consequences for rehabilitation clients and practice.

The medical model of disability

The medical model is characterized by a number of premises: an emphasis on individual autonomy rather than interaction with family and community; a view of the body as a machine needing to be "fixed"; an emphasis on diseases as entities and on "objective" assessment and diagnosis; a separation of the mind and body; and a scientific, rational and positivist approach to inquiry (Miller & Crabtree, 2005). The medical model privileges professional knowledge and authority and promotes the ideal of the "compliant" patient. It is grounded firmly in a shared understanding of "normality" and the main aim of "treatment" is to cure or restore patients to as nearly 'normal' a condition as possible. The underlying assumption is that "treatment" will result in a return to "wholeness" – an optimal level of functioning – to which all human beings should aspire but which, in reality, is not achievable for people with a disability or chronic condition. The resulting functional deficits or restrictions, which cannot be "cured", are deemed to be the inevitable and tragic consequences of the impairment (Thomas, 2004).

The individual personal tragedy model of disability

In this way, disability came to be perceived as an individual personal tragedy that required 'a process of psychological adjustment deemed necessary to enable the person to come to terms with their deficits' (Hammell, 2006, p. 58). This process was articulated in a number of stage theories of adaptation and adjustment, which required the individual to pass through recognizable phases of shock, grief, denial, anger and depression (Oliver, 2004). Failure of disabled people to achieve rehabilitation goals could then be interpreted as the individual's failure to adjust to an impairment. Such reasoning on the part of professionals leaves the rehabilitation process unchallenged and practitioners uncritically secure in their professional roles. As Hammell (2006) suggests, there is clearly a place for the medical model in an acute care delivery system, for example when an individual has a torn cruciate ligament and there is a legitimate hope of full restoration of "normal" function. However, 'intervention under such circumstances might reasonably be labeled as "treatment" performed *by* someone *to* someone else but it cannot be called rehabilitation' (Hammell, 2006, p. 59). As a result of a medicalized conception of disability, many rehabilitation practitioners and researchers equate chronic illness with disability, and disabled people become perceived as permanent "patients" (Goble, 2004). In contrast, although people with physical and mental disability and chronic conditions periodically experience physiological consequences related to their impairments or condition that require medical attention, many regard their health as excellent (Wilcock, 1998).

The ideology of independence

The medical model of disability has also given rise to an ideology of independence. This ideology equates independence in terms of self-care activities rather than the ability to take control and make decisions about one's life. There is an assumption that independence is a universally valued goal, but this is not substantiated by research evidence (Reindal, 1999). However, this preoccupation with physical independence continues to be reflected in rehabilitation practice, where a person's functional capability (or more often incapacity) is assessed using scales and tools that measure performance against "normative" standards. The main aim of rehabilitation programs is to reduce the gap, as much as possible, between the individual's performance and the 'normative' standard.

The principle of autonomy is pervasive in Western ethical, political and educational philosophy and characterizes independence as the ability to govern oneself without outside domination (Sim, 1998). This principle has been criticized by feminists and communitarian theorists as being an ideologically constructed "norm" that does not represent the reality of *inter*dependence experienced by people in the contexts of their lives. The notion of control has given rise to revised interpretations of such terms as self-government, self-rule, self-determination and self-advocacy. The notion of control in principle opens up the possibility of choosing to rely on the judgments or assistance of others in situations where we ourselves may lack the necessary information, knowledge or capability to make a reflective choice or take action (Reindal, 1999).

The biopsychosocial model

The biopsychosocial model was first proposed by Engel (1977) as a holistic alternative to the prevailing biomedical model that dominated medicine in industrialized societies. This model seeks to integrate the biological, psychological and social consequences of disability or chronic illness. According to Engel (1977), this model is both a philosophy of clinical care and a practical clinical guide. Borrell-Carrio *et al.* (2004) suggest that the biopsychosocial model is 'philosophically a way of understanding how suffering, disease, and illness are affected by multiple levels of organization, from the societal to the molecular' (p. 576). In this sense, this model has formed the theoretical foundation for the *International Classification of Functioning and Disability* (ICF) (WHO, 2001). At a practical level, 'it is a way of understanding the patient's subjective experience as an essential contributor to accurate diagnosis, health outcomes, and humane care' (Borrell-Carrio *et al.*, 2004, p. 576). Critics of this model argue that it continues to privilege the health care professionals' role and perspective, and advocate, as an alternative approach, a client-centered model of practice (Bartz, 1999).

International Classification of Functioning, Disability and Health (ICF)

The World Health Organization (WHO) published the *International Classification of Impairments, Disabilities and Handicaps* (ICIDH) in 1980. The ICIDH identified the consequences of diseases and disorders at the level of the body (impairment), the person (disability) and the person as a social being (handicap). The ICIDH definitions caused 'widespread disenchantment among disabled people and their organizations, as well as criticism from mainstream medical researchers' (Barnes & Mercer, 2003, p. 15). These criticisms focused on the biophysiological interpretation of "normality" embedded in the definitions and the clear linkages established between "disability" and "handicap". These implicit assumptions were seen as privileging medical and rehabilitation interventions in the treatment of primarily social and economic disadvantages, and representing the environment as 'neutral' (Barnes & Mercer, 2003). These criticisms caused the WHO to undergo major revisions of the ICIDH and resulted in the *International Classification of Functioning and Disability* (ICF) (WHO, 2001). The influence of the social model of disability on the ICF (also known as the ICIDH-2) can be seen in the acknowledgement that people interact with their environments. The ICF is based on the biopsychosocial model and the assumption that functioning, activity and participation are influenced by a myriad of environmental factors (Barnes & Mercer, 2003) that make up the physical, social and attitudinal environment in which people live and conduct their lives. The concept of disability in the ICF serves as an umbrella term for impairments, activity limitations or participation restrictions. The definition of impairment continues to focus on problems in body function or structure, such as a significant deviation or loss and activity limitations focused on difficulties in executing a task or action. Participation is defined as 'an individual's involvement in life situations in relation to the other ICF concepts (Health Conditions, Body Functions and Structure, Activities, and Contextual Factors)' and participation restrictions are conceived as 'the problems an individual may have in the manner or extent of involvement in life situations' (WHO, 2002, p. 10).

The WHO (2002) claims that the ICF can be used to study the impact of health and health states, provide a common language in research and provision of services, identify specific individual needs, structure outcome measures and facilitate planning of services and comparison of services across countries, disciplines, services and time through the use of a systematic coding scheme. For these reasons the ICF approach seems to hold considerable promise; however, as Hammell (2006) warns, the ICF's primary purpose remains 'to classify differences and deviations from assumed norms in every area of human life' (p. 26) and as such it is problematic. It continues to retain individualistic medical notions of disability and the linkages with impairment (Hurst, 2000) and this makes possible the unwelcome and inappropriate control of disabled people's lives by various medical and health care professions (Hammell, 2006). The issue is not to denigrate the importance of health care services to disabled people but to recognize the need to challenge the authority of professionals to make decisions that have nothing to do with medicine, such as assessing quality of life, monitoring parking permits and motor vehicle licenses, and determining who is capable of employment (Swain *et al.*, 2004; Hammell, 2006). The ICF enables professionals to code, categorize and compile statistics about people with disabilities and chronic conditions. Used judiciously and with this purpose in mind it offers new possibilities for a sociological–medical analysis of disablement (Barnes & Mercer, 2003). However, concerns have been raised (Wade & Haligan, 2003; Hammell, 2006) that the ICF is premised on "expert" assessment; that it is not an assessment tool that embodies client-centered approaches to service delivery nor one that incorporates self-appraisal of quality of life. In addition, Hammell (2004a) points out that the ICF was not developed in the context of occupational therapy and physical therapy and warns against the enthusiastic, uncritical adoption of the ICF as a framework for occupational therapy and physical therapy research, practice or curriculum development.

Quality of life as overall goal of rehabilitation

The notion of control has been shown to be integral to perceptions of quality of life (Johnstone, 2001) and it is generally agreed that quality of life is the ultimate goal of rehabilitation (Pain *et al.*, 1998; Hammell, 2006). However, a common definition of quality of life has proved difficult to establish, despite considerable theoretical discussion and research. It is generally recognized that quality of life is a multidimensional construct encompassing both objective and subjective evaluations of physical, material, social and emotional well-being, together with personal development and purposeful activity, all weighted by a unique set of personal values (Johnstone, 2001). Because there is no consensus among researchers and rehabilitation professionals about what quality of life means in the context of disability and chronic conditions, there is no agreement about how or whether measurement of it is possible or indeed if it should be attempted by the rehabilitation professions (Dijkers, 1999; Hammell, 2004a). Until recently, the majority of research has explored the objective dimensions of quality of life, using primarily quantitative research approaches such as rating scales and questionnaires, with the purpose of comparing levels of health-related quality of life between groups or before and after events or interventions (Post *et al.*, 1998). Concerns have been raised that the standardized research instruments used (for example World Health Organization, 2004), and the interpretation of data and results, inevitably reflect the researcher's beliefs, values and attitudes towards the experience of living with disability and chronic conditions (Dijkers, 1999) and reinforce the dominant models of disability, such as the medical and personal tragedy models (Swain & French, 2000).

Despite quality of life being consistently articulated as the overall goal of rehabilitation, there is little research evidence available to support the effectiveness or value of rehabilitation in promoting quality of life. This may partly be due to methodological issues associated with quality of life research (Dijkers, 1999). However, other authors suggest that some of the difficulty arises from the assumption that quality of life is a static construct (Gill, 2001) and a general neglect of the subjective evaluation of quality of life (Dijkers, 1999; Hammell, 2004b).

In addition, research (Woodend *et al.*, 1997; Albrecht & Devlieger, 1999) has demonstrated the discrepancy between the objective (that is, the researcher's) assessment of quality of life and the subjective (that is, the client's) satisfaction with that life (Hammell, 2004b). As Hammell (2006) suggests, 'how a researcher or clinician attempts to measure "quality of life" [may] reveal more about their own values, priorities and fundamental orientation to life than it does about the quality of life perceived by people whose lives are ostensibly being studied' (p. 139). There is an increasing recognition of the need to involve people with experience of disability and chronic conditions in the evaluation of quality of life. This recognition has prompted many authors (for example Dijkers, 1999; Johnstone, 2001; Hammell & Carpenter, 2004) to argue that the subjective experience of quality of life requires the implementation of rigorous qualitative and mixed methods research approaches. Hammell (2006) reflects her belief that the quality of life can only be appraised by the person whose life it is, when she proposes that the term "quality of life" be simply conceptualized 'as the experience of a life worth living' (p. 138).

The social model of disability

The social model of disability arose from the publication of *Fundamental Principles of Disability* by the Union of Physically Impaired Against Segregation (UPIAS) in 1976. This model presented an interpretation of disability not as an individual and personal characteristic but as a shared and collective responsibility (Johnstone, 2001). The fundamental assertion was that society disables people who have impairments: 'In our view it is society which disables physically impaired people. Disability is something imposed on top of our impairments by the way we are unnecessarily isolated and excluded from full participation in society' (UPIAS, 1976 p. 14). Thus, this model brought to the forefront issues of structural and personal barriers created by society, and recognized the need for the participation of disabled people in decision-making and the limitations of professional expertise. This analysis is built on a clear distinction rather than a causal link between impairment and disability. A medical definition of impairment was adopted as, 'lacking part or all of a limb, or having a defective limb, organ or mechanism of the body' (UPIAS cited by Thomas, 2004, p. 25). Disability was defined variously as: 'A condition in which people with impairments are discriminated against, segregated and denied full participative citizenship' (Swain *et al.*, 2003), and: the loss or limitation of opportunities which prevent people who have impairments from taking part in the activities of the community on an equal level with others due to physical and social barriers (Swain *et al.*, 2004).

A number of criticisms have been levelled at the social model of disability over the ensuing years. This model appears to ignore, or is unable to deal adequately with, the realities of impairment. Attempts to separate the experience of disability and impairment, and to insist that physical differences and restrictions are entirely socially created, contradicts an individual's everyday experiences (Barnes & Mercer, 2003). It has been suggested also that the definition of impairment excludes and marginalizes some groups, for example people who describe themselves as 'mental health system survivors' and those with learning difficulties, and that 'it has tended to downplay the potential for considerable variation in experience of both disability and impairment across the disabled population' (Barnes & Mercer, 2003, p. 70). A related criticism focuses on the issue of "otherness" and argues that it is not the physical and environmental barriers people face, but the way society's values position disabled people as "other" (Oliver, 2004). However, the social model's definition of disability has made it possible to identify the range, form and types of discrimination that make the world a difficult place for disabled people and to differentiate these from impairment issues (Thomas, 2004).

The social model of disability is reflected in recently developed theories of occupational therapy, for example occupational performance (Canadian Association of Occupational Therapists, 2000), and in physical therapy, for example the movement continuum theory (Cott et al., 1995). Both these examples acknowledge the importance of social, cultural, economic, political and legal environments as well as the physical. In general, rehabilitation professionals remain firmly entrenched in a medical model of service delivery that is focused upon individualized health care services (Crichton & Jongbloed, 1998; Hammell, 2003), but there are examples of practitioners who have clearly positioned their research and discussions about practice in relation to the social model of disability (Marquis & Jackson, 2000; Hawkins & Stewart, 2002; Kemp, 2002; Lund & Nygard, 2004). This issue of 'positioning oneself' as the researcher in terms of theoretical influences was alluded to earlier in this chapter and will be addressed in more detail in Chapter 7.

Client-centered practice

A review of the rehabilitation literature (for example Law, 1998) clearly indicates that the occupational therapy profession has been debating the concept of client-centered practice for over two decades. Client-centered practice has been recognized as a key professional behavior in physical therapy (MacDonald et al., 2001). However, there has been little consistent discussion to date in the physical therapy literature. During the same period of time an increased prevalence of chronic disability, increasingly sophisticated and well-informed health consumers, and increasing demands for health care practitioners to be accountable have prompted governments to take a more client-oriented approach to health service delivery (for example Department of Health 2001, 2005). In addition, reflective of the underlying philosophy of individualism that is dominant in Western cultures, the principle of respect for autonomy (Beauchamp & Childress, 2001) has given rise to the ethical and legal imperative of informed consent (Sim, 1998). This requires at least a degree of shared information and decision-making between clients and service providers, favouring active engagement over passivity (Hammell, 2006). Client-centered practice has been described as a collaborative approach to practice that encourages client autonomy, choice and control and that respects clients' abilities and supports their right to enact these choices (Sumsion & Law, 2006). Similarly, Law (1998) defined it as 'An approach to service which embraces a philosophy of respect for, and partnership with, people receiving services' (p. 3).

In the current climate of political and ethical imperatives and professional standards, client-centered practice is no longer a practice approach to be discussed theoretically 'as a mode of service to which professions might aspire if and when they choose' (Hammell, 2006, p. 154). However, relatively little research (for example Guadagnoli & Ward, 1998; Marquis & Jackson, 2000; Ford et al., 2003; Blank, 2004) has been conducted exploring the meaning and experience of client-centered practice from the client's perspective. In fact, some authors (for example Abberley, 2004; Dalley, 1999; Martone, 2001) suggest that professional claims of client-centered rehabilitation practice are more rhetorical than based in reality. However, research does suggest that increasing client participation and control in the rehabilitation process has been linked to favorable outcomes (MacLeod & MacLeod, 1996; Albrecht & Devlieger, 1999; Marquis & Jackson, 2000; Lorig et al., 2001; Ford et al., 2003) and that clients place more importance in the interpersonal qualities and communication skills of health professionals than in their technical skills (Gage, 1999; MacLean et al., 2000; French, 2004).

Research has also indicated that clients want to receive services that are based on evidence that demonstrates their effectiveness (Ford et al., 2003). However, in rehabilitation, where clients are attempting to assimilate the effects of injury and chronic illness into the continuum of their lives, therapy decisions based on the best available evidence derived from predominantly quantitative research may not correspond with therapy practice that focuses on the client's wishes and preferences, short- and long-term goals, their social support and the impact of chronic disability on their lifestyle. Tensions exist between the philosophies of client-centered practice and evidence-based practice that require negotiation in the delivery of rehabilitation services (Hammell, 2001).

Evidence-based rehabilitation practice

Evidence-based practice (EBP) is 'a significant movement of fundamental importance in the delivery of health care throughout the developing world' (Bithell, 2000, p. 58). It represents an expansion of the concept of evidence-based medicine to encompass more aspects of health care, including rehabilitation (Law, 2002). The rehabilitation disciplines have willingly subscribed to the evidence-based movement and its culture of accountability (Carpenter, 2004), and recognize that if 'evidence-based practice can be incorporated into the practitioner's repertoire, the professions will see a shift toward a more analytical, certain, and ultimately effective clinical practice' (Law, 2002, p. 8). Unfortunately, earlier definitions of EBP (Sackett et al., 1996) promoted the idea of a hierarchy of evidence that privileged randomized control trials (RCTs) as a sort of "gold standard." This association of research evidence with experimental research approaches has served to restrict the sort of questions it has been possible to ask and the sort of issues it has made possible to investigate (Hyde, 2004). A more recent and broader iteration of EBP incorporates three dimensions – the conscientious and judicious use of relevant and current research evidence, clinical expertise and patient values and preferences – into clinical decision-making (Sackett et al., 2000).

Most rehabilitation professionals recognize that the complex issues inherent in rehabilitation practice entail far more than a wholesale application of research to practice, because even best evidence can lead to bad practice if applied uncritically. In addition, authors seldom link the terms evidence-based practice and patient/client-centered practice (Benzing, 2000). This is not surprising given that the concept of evidence-based practice is essentially an impairment or disease-oriented and practitioner-centered approach (Benzing, 2000; Miller & Crabtree, 2005). Sweeney *et al.* (1998) observed that EBP continues to focus on the clinician's interpretation and application of the evidence to intervention decisions, and diminishes the importance of human relationships and the role of the patient. This focus can be seen quite clearly in the broader definition of EBP (Sackett *et al.*, 2000) cited earlier, where the assumption is that practitioners will incorporate the evidence and patient perspectives in making a clinical decision. There is, however, an increasing call in medicine and rehabilitation to strengthen the client-centeredness of EBP (Sweeney *et al.*, 1998; Benzing, 2000; Holm, 2005; Miller & Crabtree, 2005; Hammell, 2006). Such 'patient-centered clinical research' (Sackett *et al.*, 2000, p. 1) must include greater methodological diversity, notably by including qualitative research (Bithell, 2000; Ritchie, 2001; Gibson & Martin, 2003; Hammell & Carpenter, 2004; Johnson & Waterfield, 2004; Blair & Robertson, 2005; Miller & Crabtree, 2005) and developing more effective approaches to synthesizing the evidence that is available (Benzing, 2000).

Defining rehabilitation

The way we, as rehabilitation professionals, define rehabilitation and related concepts, and use terminology reveals a great deal about the, often taken-for-granted, professional and personal values and beliefs we hold about our role and responsibilities and the client–professional interaction in the rehabilitation process. As qualitative researchers, it is essential that we reflect and articulate the theoretical, professional and personal influences we bring to the research endeavor. With this in mind, we think that it is important for us to make our use of terminology and concepts as clear as possible throughout the book. Hence, our decision to use double quotation marks to denote terms we consider controversial when used in certain contexts. There has been considerable debate about the definitions and language used in relation to disability and impairment (see, for example, Johnstone, 2001; Barnes & Mercer, 2003; Finkelstein, 2004; Hammell, 2006). Much of this debate has focused on the use of the terms "disabled people" and "people with disabilities". By adopting the definition of disability as representing the physical, political, economic, legal, social and cultural experiences of living with an impairment (Hammell, 2006) we align ourselves with the social model of disability. Disability theorists argue that the term "disabled people" is preferable to "people with disabilities" because it better reflects 'the ways social barriers affect life chances' (Barnes & Mercer, 2003, p. 18) as opposed to representing disability as an individual characteristic. We will use the term "disabled people" throughout this book.

Merriam-Webster's Online Medical Dictionary (2005) defines rehabilitation as 'the physical restoration of a sick or disabled person by therapeutic measures and re-education to participate in activities of a normal life within the limitations of the person's physical disability'. This definition clearly reflects the individual or medical model of disability characterized by the assumptions of "normalization", physical independence as an aim of the rehabilitative process and the disabled person's adaptation to a pre-existing environment. For the purpose of this book we will adopt the more comprehensive definition of rehabilitation as 'a process of enabling someone to live well with an impairment in the context of his or her own environment and, as such, requires a complex, individually tailored approach' (Hammell, 2006, p. 8). The brief overview of the models of disability and approaches to health care delivery provided in this chapter highlights the theoretical contexts within which rehabilitation services are delivered and the different ways that rehabilitation can be defined. The following chapter will explore the philosophical systems that form the foundation of qualitative research and the assumptions that characterize qualitative approaches.

References

Abberley, P. (2004) A critique of professional support and intervention. In: J. Swain, S. French, C. Barnes & C. Thomas (eds), *Disabling Barriers – Enabling Environments* (2nd edn, pp. 239–244). Thousand Oaks, Calif., Sage.

Albrecht, G.L. & Devlieger, P.J. (1999) The disability paradox: high quality life against all odds. *Social Science & Medicine*, 48, 977–988.

Bailey, D.M. & Jackson, J.M. (2003) Qualitative data analysis: challenges and dilemmas related to theory and method. *American Journal of Occupational Therapy*, 57 (1), 57–65.

Ballinger, C. (2004) Writing up rigour: representing and evaluating good scholarship in qualitative research. *British Journal of Occupational Therapy*, 67 (12), 540–546.

Barnes, C. & Mercer, G. (2003) *Disability*. Oxford, Blackwell Publishing.

Bartz, R. (1999) Beyond the biopsychosocial model: new approaches to doctor–patient interactions. *Journal of Family Practice*, 48, 601–607.

Baum, C. & Christiansen, C. (1997) The occupational therapy context: philosophy – principles – practice. In: C. Christiansen & C. Baum (eds), *Occupational Therapy: Enabling Function and Well-being* (2nd edn, pp. 28–45). Thorofare, NJ, Slack.

Beauchamp, T.L. & Childress, J.F. (2001) *Principles of Biomedical Ethics* (5th edn). New York, Oxford University Press.

Becker, H.S., Geer, B., Hughes, E.C. & Strauss, A.L. (1961) *Boys in White: Student Culture in Medical School*. Chicago, University of Chicago Press.

Benzing, J. (2000) Bridging the gap. The separate worlds of evidence-based medicine and patient-centered medicine. *Patient Education and Counselling*, 39, 17–25.

Bithell, C. (2000) Evidence-based physiotherapy: some thoughts on 'best evidence'. *Physiotherapy*, 86 (2), 58–61.

Blair, S. & Robertson, L.J. (2005) Hard complexities – soft complexities: an exploration of philosophical positions related to evidence in occupational therapy. *British Journal of Occupational Therapy*, 68 (6), 269–276.

Blank, A. (2004) Clients' experience of partnership with occupational therapists in community mental health. *British Journal of Occupational Therapy*, 67 (3), 118–124.

Bloch, M. (2004) A discourse that disciplines, governs and regulates: the National Research Council's report on scientific research in education. *Qualitative Inquiry*, 10 (1), 96–110.

Bogdan, R.C. & Biklen, S.K. (1998) *Qualitative Research for Education: an Introduction to Theory and Methods* (3rd edn). Boston, Allyn & Bacon.

Borrell-Carrio, F., Suchman, A.L. & Epstein, R.M. (2004) The biopsychosocial model 25 years later: principles, practice and scientific inquiry. *Annals of Family Medicine*, 2 (6), 576–582.

Canadian Association of Occupational Therapists (2000) *Enabling Occupation: An Occupational Therapy Perspective* (2nd edn). Ottawa, Canadian Association of Occupational Therapists.

Carpenter, C. (1994) The experience of spinal cord injury: the individual's perspective – implications for rehabilitation practice. *Physical Therapy*, 74 (7), 614–629.

Carpenter, C. (1997) Conducting qualitative research in physiotherapy: a methodological example. *Physiotherapy*, 83 (10), 547–552.

Carpenter, C. (2004) The contribution of qualitative research to evidence-based practice. In: K.W. Hammell & C. Carpenter (eds), *Qualitative Research in Evidence-based Rehabilitation* (pp. 1–13). Edinburgh, Churchill Livingstone.

Corbet, B. (2000) Bully pulpit: bound for glory. *New Mobility*, 11 (83), 4–5.

Cott, C., Finch, E. & Gasner, D. (1995) The movement continuum theory of physical therapy. *Physiotherapy Canada*, 47 (2), 87–95.

Creswell, J. (1998) *Qualitative Inquiry and Research Designs: Choosing Among Five Traditions*. Thousand Oaks, Calif., Sage.

Crichton, A. & Jongbloed, L. (1998) *Disability and Social Policy in Canada*. North York, Ont., Captus.

Dalley, J. (1999) Evaluation of clinical practice: is a client-centered approach compatible with professional issues? *Physiotherapy*, 85 (9), 491–497.

Davidson, I. & Waters, K. (2000) Physiotherapists working with stroke patients: a national survey. *Physiotherapy*, 86 (2), 69–80.

Denzin, N.K., & Lincoln, Y.S. (2005) Introduction: the discipline and practice of qualitative research. In: N.K. Denzin & Y.S. Lincoln (eds), *The Sage Handbook of Qualitative Research* (3rd edn, pp. 1–32). Thousand Oaks, Calif., Sage.

Department of Health (2001) *The Expert Patient: a New Approach to Chronic Disease Management for the Twenty-first Century*. London, Department of Health.

Department of Health (2005) *Creating a Patient-led NHS: Delivering the NHS Improvement Plan*. London, Department of Health.

De Souza, L. (1998) Editorial – theories about therapies are underdeveloped. *Physiotherapy Research International*, 3 (3), iv–vi.

Dijkers, M. (1999) Measuring quality of life: methodological issues. *American Journal of Physical Medicine and Rehabilitation*, 78, 286–300.

Dyck, I. (2000) Working with theory in qualitative research. In: K.W. Hammell, C. Carpenter & I. Dyck (eds), *Using Qualitative Research: a Practical Introduction for Occupational and Physical Therapists* (pp. 85–95). Edinburgh, Churchill Livingstone.

Engel, G. (1977) The need for a new medical model: a challenge for biomedicine. *Science*, 196 (4286), 129–135.

Fealy, G.M. (1997) The theory–practice relationship in nursing: an exploration of the contemporary discourse. *Journal of Advanced Nursing*, 25, 1061–1069.

Field, P.A. & Morse, J.A. (1985) *Nursing Research: the Application of Qualitative Approaches*. Thousand Oaks, Calif., Sage.

Finkelstein, V. (2004) Representing disability. In: J. Swain, S. French, C. Barnes & C. Thomas (eds), *Disabling Barriers – Enabling Environments* (2nd edn, pp. 13–20). Thousand Oaks, Calif., Sage.

Ford, S., Schofield, T. & Hope, T. (2003) What are the ingredients for a successful evidence-based patient choice consultation? a qualitative study. *Social Science & Medicine, 56*, 589–602.

French, S. (2004) Enabling relationships in therapy practice. In: J. Swain, J. Clark & S. French (eds), *Enabling Relationships in Health and Social Care: a Guide for Therapists* (pp. 95–107). Oxford, Butterworth Heinemann.

Gage, M. (1999) Physical disabilities: meeting the challenge of client-centered practice. In: T. Sumsion (ed.), *Client-centered Practice in Occupational Therapy*, (pp. 89–101). Edinburgh, Churchill Livingstone.

Geertz, C. (1973) *The Interpretation of Cultures: Selected Essays*. New York, Basic Books.

Geertz, C. (1983) *Local Knowledge: Further Essays in Interpretive Anthropology*. New York, Basic Books.

Gibson, B.E. & Martin, D.K. (2003) Qualitative research and evidence-based physiotherapy practice. *Physiotherapy, 89* (6), 350–358.

Gill, C.J. (2001) Divided understandings: the social experience of disability. In: G.L. Albrecht, K.D. Seelman & M. Bury (eds) *Handbook of Disability Studies* (pp. 351–372). Thousand Oaks, Calif., Sage.

Glaser, B.G. & Strauss, A.L. (1967) *The Discovery of Grounded Theory: Strategies for Qualitative Research*. Chicago, Aldine.

Goble, C. (2004) Dependence, independence and normality. In: J. Swain, S. French, C. Barnes & C. Thomas (eds). *Disabling Barriers – Enabling Environments* (2nd edn, pp. 41–46). Thousand Oaks, Calif., Sage.

Guadagnoli, E. & Ward, P. (1998) Patient participation in decision-making. *Social Science and Medicine, 47* (3), 329–339.

Hammell, K.W. (2001) Using qualitative research to inform the client-centered evidence-based practice of occupational therapy. *British Journal of Occupational Therapy, 64* (5), 228–234.

Hammell, K.W. (2003) Changing institutional environments to enable occupation among people with severe physical impairments. In: L. Letts, P. Rigby & D. Stewart (eds), *Using Environments to Enable Occupational Performance* (pp. 35–53). Thorofare, NJ, Slack.

Hammell, K.W. (2004a) Deviating from the norm: a sceptical interrogation of the classificatory practices of the ICF. *British Journal of Occupational Therapy, 67* (9), 408–411.

Hammell, K.W. (2004b) Exploring quality of life following spinal cord injury: a review and critique. *Spinal Cord, 42*, 491–502.

Hammell, K.W. (2006) *Perspectives on Disability and Rehabilitation: Contesting Assumptions, Challenging Practice*. Edinburgh, Churchill Livingstone Elsevier.

Hammell, K.W. & Carpenter, C. (2004) *Qualitative Research in Evidence-based Rehabilitation*. Edinburgh, Churchill Livingstone.

Hammell, K.W. Carpenter, C. & Dyck, I. (2000) *Using Qualitative Research: a Practical Introduction for Occupational and Physical Therapists*. London, Churchill Livingstone.

Hawkins, R. & Stewart, S. (2002) Changing rooms: the impact of adaptations on the meaning of home for a disabled person and the role of occupational therapists in the process. *British Journal of Occupational Therapy, 65* (2), 81–87.

Holm, S. (2005) Justifying patient self-management – evidence based medicine or the primacy of the first person perspective. *Medicine, Health Care and Philosophy, 8* (2), 159–164.

Howe, K.R. (2004) A critique of experimentalism. *Qualitative Inquiry, 10* (1), 42–61.

Hurst, R. (2000) To revise or not to revise? *Disability and Society, 15* (7), 1083–1087.

Hyde, P. (2004) Fool's gold: examining the use of gold standards in the production of research evidence. *British Journal of Occupational Therapy*, *67* (2), 89–94.

Johnson, R. & Waterfield, J. (2004) Making words count: the value of qualitative research. *Physiotherapy Research International*, *9* (3), 121–131.

Johnstone, D. (2001) *An Introduction to Disability Studies* (2nd edn, pp. 112–122). London, David Fulton Publishers.

Kemp, L. (2002) Why are some people's needs unmet? *Disability & Society*, *17* (2), 205–218.

Law, M. (ed.) (1998) *Client-centered Occupational Therapy*. Thorofare, NJ, Slack.

Law, M. (ed.) (2002) *Evidence-based Rehabilitation: a Guide to Practice*. Thorofare, NJ, Slack.

Lorig, K., Sobel, D.S., Ritter, P.L., Laurent, D. & Hobbs, M. (2001) Effect of a self-management program on patients with chronic disease. *Effective Clinical Practice*, *4*, 256–562.

Lund, M.L. & Nygard, L. (2004) Occupational life in the home environment: the experiences of people with disabilities. *The Canadian Journal of Occupational Therapy*, *71* (4), 243–251.

MacDonald, C., Houghton, P., Cox, P. & Bartlett, D. (2001) Consensus on physical therapy professional behaviors. *Physiotherapy Canada*, *53* (3), 212–218.

MacLean, N., Pound, P., Wolfe, C. & Rudd, A. (2000) Qualitative analysis of stroke patients' motivation for rehabilitation. *British Medical Journal*, *7268* (28 Oct.), 1051–1054.

MacLeod, G. & MacLeod, L. (1996) Evaluation of client and staff satisfaction with a goal planning project implemented with people with spinal cord injuries. *Spinal Cord*, *34*, 525–530.

Malinowski, B. (1922) *Argonauts of the Western Pacific*. London, Routledge & Kegan Paul.

Marquis, R. & Jackson, R. (2000) Quality of life and quality service relationships: experiences of people with disabilities. *Disability & Society*, *15* (3), 411–425.

Martone, M. (2001) Decision-making issues in the rehabilitation process. *Hastings Center Report*, *31* (2), 36–41.

Merriam-Webster Online Medical Dictionary (2005) Retrieved 10 April 2007 from: http://www.nlm.nih.gov/medline plus/mplusdictionary.html

Merriam-Webster Online Dictionary (2006) Retrieved 26 February 2007 from: http://www.m-w.com/

Miller, W.L. & Crabtree, B.F. (2005) Clinical research. In: N.K. Denzin & Y.S. Lincoln (eds) *The Sage Handbook of Qualitative Research* (3rd edn, pp. 605–639). Thousand Oaks, Calif., Sage.

Oliver, M. (2004) If I had a hammer: the social model in action. In: J. Swain, S. French, C. Barnes & C. Thomas (eds), *Disabling Barriers – Enabling Environments* (2nd edn, pp. 7–12). Thousand Oaks, Calif., Sage.

Pain, K., Dunn, M., Anderson, G., Darrah, J. & Kratochville, M. (1998) Quality of life: what does it mean in rehabilitation? *Journal of Rehabilitation*, *64* (2), 5–11.

Post, M., de Witte, L., van Asbek, F., van Dijk, A. & Schrijvers, A. (1998) Predictors of health status and life satisfaction in spinal cord injury. *Archives of Physical Medicine and Rehabilitation*, *78*, 395–402.

Reindal, S.M. (1999) Independence, dependence, interdependence: some reflections on the subject and personal autonomy. *Disability & Society*, *14* (3), 353–367.

Richardson, B. (1999) Professional development: 2. Professional knowledge and situated learning in the workplace. *Physiotherapy*, *85* (9), 467–473.

Ritchie, J. (2001) Not everything can be reduced to numbers. In: C. Berglund (ed.), *Health Research*. Oxford, Oxford University Press.

Robertson, V. (1994) A quantitative analysis of research in physical therapy. *Physical Therapy*, *75* (4), 313–321.

Roskell, C., Hewison, A. & Wildman, S. (1998) The theory–practice gap and physiotherapy in the UK: insights from the nursing experience. *Physiotherapy Theory and Practice*, *14*, 223–233.

Sackett, D., Richardson, W., Rosenberg, W. & Haynes, R. (1996) *Evidence-based Medicine*. Edinburgh, Churchill Livingstone.

Sackett, D., Strauss, S., Richardson, W., Rosenberg, W. & Haynes, R. (2000) *Evidence-based Medicine: How to Practice and Teach EBP* (2nd edn). Edinburgh, Churchill Livingstone.

Shepard, K.F., Jensen, G.M., Schmoll, B.J., Hack, L.M. & Gwyer, J. (1993) Alternative approaches to research in physical therapy: positivism and phenomenology. *Physical Therapy*, *73* (2), 88–97.

Sim, J. (1998) Respect for autonomy: issues in neurological rehabilitation. *Clinical Rehabilitation*, *12*, 3–10.

Sumsion, T. & Law, M. (2006) A review of evidence on the conceptual elements informing client-centered practice. *Canadian Journal of Occupational Therapy*, *73* (3), 153–162.

Swain, J. & French, S. (2000) Towards an affirmation model of disability. *Disability & Society*, *1* (4), 569–582.

Swain, J., French, S. & Cameron, C. (2003) *Controversial Issues in a Disabling Society*. Buckingham, Open University Press.

Swain, J., French, S., Barnes, C. & Thomas, C. (2004) *Disabling Barriers – Enabling Environments* (2nd edn). London, Sage.

Sweeney, K.G., MacAuley, D. & Gray, D.P. (1998) Personal significance: the third dimension. *Lancet*, *351*, 134–136.

Thomas, C. (2004) Disability and impairment. In: J. Swain, S. French, C. Barnes & C. Thomas (eds), *Disabling Barriers – Enabling Environments* (2nd edn, pp. 21–27). Thousand Oaks, Calif., Sage.

Union of Physically Impaired Against Segregation (1976) *Fundamental Principles of Disability*. London, Union of Physically Impaired Against Segregation.

Wade, D. & Haligan, P. (2003) New wine in old bottles: the WHO ICF as an explanatory model of human behavior. *Clinical Rehabilitation*, *17* (4), 349–354.

Walker, M.F., Drummond, A.E.R., Gatt, J. & Sackley, C.M. (2000) Occupational therapy for stroke patients: a survey of current practice. *British Journal of Occupational Therapy*, *63* (8), 367–372.

Wilcock, A.A. (1998) Occupation for health. *British Journal of Occupational Therapy*, *61* (8), 340–345.

Woodend, A.K., Nair, R.C. & Tang, A.S. (1997) Definition of life quality from a patient versus health care professional perspective. *International Journal of Rehabilitation Research*, *20*, 71–80.

World Health Organization (1980) *International Classification of Impairments, Disabilities and Handicaps*. Geneva, World Health Organization.

World Health Organization (2001) *International Classification of Functioning, Disability and Health*. Geneva, World Health Organization.

World Health Organization (2002) *Towards a Common Language for Functioning, Disability and Health: ICF Beginners' Guide* (pdf document). Retrieved 12 March 2007 from: http://www3.who.int/icf/icftemplate.cfm

World Health Organization (2004) *Quality of Life (WHOQOL)*. Geneva, World Health Organization.

Chapter 2

WHY CHOOSE QUALITATIVE RESEARCH IN REHABILITATION?

Introduction

There are many reasons for the good fit between qualitative research and the contemporary issues facing occupational therapists and physical therapists and their rehabilitation clients. In this chapter we describe the philosophical assumptions and theoretical perspectives that characterize qualitative research and begin to explore its potential to illuminate the complex issues associated with client-centered and evidence-based practice. As stated in Chapter 1, qualitative research is well suited to answer questions that ask *what* particular experiences are like and *how* people create meaning from their circumstances. These types of questions are appropriate for topics where little is known from the client's point of view, and much depends on how knowledge is created, and for whose benefit.

As the demand for evidence to substantiate physical therapy and occupational therapy practice continues, a concurrent tension exists between an increasingly knowledgeable, Internet-savvy public and the authority assumed by health care professionals. How are theories developed? Is the evidence that we create through research relevant to outcomes that matter to clients? How is it that physical therapists and occupational therapists come to know what matters to people who are disabled or live with a chronic health condition? Qualitative research has a role to play in identifying the concepts that help us understand people's lives, contributing evidence to support rehabilitation theories, and linking this knowledge to existing social theories. The increased availability of community-based services highlights the importance of developing theories that emerge from and are relevant to the social, political, economic and cultural contexts in which clients live. It is important that researchers begin their inquiry process with an examination of the 'philosophical assumptions about the nature of reality (ontology), how they know what is known (epistemology), the inclusion of their values (*axiology*), and the nature in which their research emerges (*methodology*)' (Creswell *et al.*, 2007, p. 238), as these provide an intellectual scaffold for examining the unique characteristics underlying qualitative research. In this chapter we introduce key philosophical systems that have influenced qualitative research (ontology) and describe the types of knowledge that rehabilitation professionals use (epistemology) and, later in the book, we will discuss four methodological approaches common to health care research (in Chapter 4) and the *reflexivity* (axiological) issues central to conducting qualitative research (in Chapter 7).

Key philosophical systems

In Chapter 1, we explained that a profession's philosophy, which is made up of values, beliefs and principles, provides a framework from which to examine ontological and epistemological questions. Far from being academic questions, the ontological and epistemological positions that a profession and its scholars take have a powerful impact on rehabilitation discourse (Hammell, 2006). Whether explicitly written or implicitly transmitted through practice, this discourse influences students, practitioners and ultimately clients, as well as the decisions about what constitutes worthwhile research. To answer the question: 'Why choose qualitative research in rehabilitation?' it is first necessary to examine the contributions to qualitative research of three key philosophical systems: *interpretivism, constructivism* and *critical theory*, which are also known as 'theoretical paradigms and perspectives' (Denzin & Lincoln, 2005, p. 23). As with other schools of thought and processes of knowledge development, definitional variation exists among researchers and theorists. It is important to understand the similarities and differences between interpretivism, constructivism and critical theory so that researchers can select the framework that fits best with their worldview, that is, their ontological and epistemological positions, and is congruent with their research question or purpose.

Interpretivism and constructivism

Naturalistic or qualitative inquiry is the name of a reformist movement that developed in the 1960s and 1970s with the aim of challenging the positivist notion of a 'grand narrative' or single "truth" in favour of alternative, transactional knowledge focused on the concept of *multiple realities*. The philosophical approach to knowledge and inquiry of Schutz (1970) exemplifies this radical shift in thinking. For Schutz, all human action is meaningful and he was committed to the idea of knowledge generated by individuals located in the life world: the common-sense world that is taken for granted. According to Schutz (1970) the life world encompassed 'the whole sphere of everyday experiences, orientations, and actions through which individuals pursue their interests and affairs by manipulating objects, dealing with people, conceiving plans, and carrying them out' (p. 14). This common-sense reality comprised the historical and cultural elements held in common by individuals, but the manner in which these are interpreted in each individual's life depended on an individual's total experience. This totality included, for Schutz (1970), each person's 'biographical situation': their special interests, motives, desires, aspirations, religious and ideological values, through which each individual interprets what they encounter in the social world. Schutz emphasized that this world is intersubjective, that is, a world where people come into relationship with each other and try and come to terms with, or interpret, each other's actions. Whilst individuals cannot directly adopt the perspective of another individual it is possible to recognize and engage in similar experiences or actions, making it feasible to share a common interpretation of aspects of their reality.

At the core of the interpretivist approach is an interest in understanding the complex world of lived experience or life world, and a respect for the perspective of those individuals who live and interact within that world. From this perspective human action is meaningful and the goal of interpretive inquiry is the grasping or understanding of how people interpret or make meaning of social phenomena. Interpretivism is closely aligned with the philosophical concept of *hermeneutics*, which is defined as 'the methodology and principles of studying interpretation, meaning and purpose' (Dyson & Brown, 2006, p. 190). Interpretivism and hermeneutics form the philosophical underpinnings of *phenomenology* within which there are two main schools of thought: interpretive and descriptive. Researchers working within an interpretivist or hermeneutic tradition draw upon the notion of the hermeneutic interpretive circle as a method or procedure unique to the human sciences. As Schwandt (2000) explains: 'In order to understand the part (the specific sentence, utterance or act), the inquirer must grasp the whole (the complex of intentions, beliefs, and desires or the text, institutional context, practice, life style, language and so on), and vice versa' (p. 193). In interpretive phenomenology, researchers use a systematic analytic process to understand meanings that cannot be discerned through textual analysis only. In contrast, but sharing some of the processes, a descriptive approach is used in phenomenology by researchers who believe that meanings are discernible through precise and careful descriptive accounts of lived experiences that are reflected in text (Rapport, 2005).

Constructivism, on the other hand, is premised on the socially and culturally situated nature of human action and can be defined as 'an approach in social science based on an assumption that human beings construct their social reality, and that the social world cannot exist independently of human beings' (Holloway, 2005, p. 290). From a constructivist perspective, knowledge is built through increasingly nuanced reconstructions of individual and group experiences. There is no single reality that can be reduced or approximated, only multiple, constructed realities (Schwandt, 2000). This knowledge leads to "truth" claims that are situated more towards relativism, that is, away from the position that there are 'permanent, unvarying (or "foundational") standards by which truth can be universally known' (Guba & Lincoln, 2005, p. 204). Backman *et al.* (2007) exemplify a constructivist approach in their study, which describes the parenting experiences of women with inflammatory arthritis and explores the phenomena that contribute to participation in mothering. The "reality" privileged in this study is that of the women living with arthritis and participating in the occupations of motherhood rather than a singular reality arising from propositional knowledge based within a biomedical model.

Critical theory

Critical theory is situated within post-modern discourse and encompasses a range of perspectives including feminism, Marxism, post-colonialism, cultural studies and queer theory (Carspecken, 1996; Denzin & Lincoln, 2005). Kincheloe &

McLaren (2005) propose the following definition: 'a critical social theory is concerned in particular with issues of power and justice and the ways that the economy; matters of race, class and gender; ideologies; discourses; education; religion and other social institutions; and cultural dynamics interact to construct a social system' (p. 306). Critical theory differs from constructivism in that the emphasis is on concepts and practices that aim to emancipate and enlighten individuals and groups, illuminate power relations and the role of economics, and uncover the ideologies that implicitly shape people's lives. Although multiple realities are acknowledged, the interpretation of these is tempered by historical realities that differ from the more situated and relativist knowledge co-construction that is sought in constructivist approaches. For example, a researcher who is interested in how leisure participation affects health outcomes might aim to understand the meaning of leisure participation and health (constructivist) through textual analysis of the research participants' lived experiences. Alternatively, a researcher with the same general interest could focus on societal beliefs, health and leisure discourses, and accessibility issues (critical theory) that influence leisure participation for people within different income groups.

The use of critical theory approaches is increasingly applicable to knowledge development in occupational therapy and physical therapy as these professions move beyond a focus primarily on individuals to an examination of larger social systems that shape individual lives. What follows is a description of selected critical theory concepts that are relevant to current issues in rehabilitation and which inform methodological approaches such as ethnography and participatory action research.

The aim of a researcher working from a critical theory perspective is to critique the socially constructed and mediated experiences of people that may otherwise be disguised as natural or inevitable (Kincheloe & McLaren, 2005). The process of identifying a taken-for-granted phenomenon and revealing the particular social and economic processes that contribute to it is an example of *problematizing*, which is central to any critical theory. Sakellariou & Algado (2006) aptly problematize the issue of sexuality and disabled people as one of 'occupational injustice' and they suggest that its absence from occupational therapy reflects society's beliefs and attitudes that people with spinal cord injuries are asexual and thus excluded from this human dimension. The goal of *critical enlightenment* is to uncover the power relations that shape those experiences and reveal the distribution and operation of power and privilege. In rehabilitation, for example, it may seem natural that services are provided in an institutional setting but it is also a context where the control and authority of professionals, however well-meaning, are maintained and seldom questioned. For people living with serious mental health problems, the prescription of medication by physicians may be helpful for symptom management but it also positions medical knowledge as the dominant force in treatment and reinforces doctors' unexamined positions of privilege in most societies.

The concept of *critical emancipation* focuses on furthering human agency through empowerment. Lather (1991) describes this notion of empowerment as a phenomenon that occurs through analyses of 'systemic oppressive forces' (p. 4) that influence the conditions under which people live, rather than something arising from an individual sense of feeling powerful and acting assertively. Language and power are interrelated critical theory concepts that refer to the discursive power of language and its role in constructing a view of the world rather than describing exactly what is observed and experienced (Kincheloe & McLaren, 2005). Discursive power may be understood by exposing who is given a voice through being a research participant and how voices of the participants and the researchers are constructed in the text. How language, voice and power contribute to particular discourses is revealed by examining the pervasive influence of the biomedical model within physical therapy and occupational therapy curricula. Historically, professional voices have dominated to the extent that the client or patient's perspective was absent in textbooks (see Crepeau *et al.*, 2003), which in turn influenced how problems or issues were named and understood. The notion that clients are the experts in their own lives, now widely accepted, arose in part from the emergence of alternative discourses, such as the independent living movement and, within mental health, the recovery paradigm and the advent of disability studies.

Hegemony and *ideology* are critical theory concepts that may initially seem foreign or irrelevant to occupational therapy and physical therapy, and they certainly require more than a quick reading to grasp. O'Sullivan *et al.* (1994) define hegemony as 'the ability in certain historical periods of the dominant classes to exercise social and cultural leadership, and by these means – rather than by direct coercion of subordinate classes – to maintain their power over the economic, political and cultural direction of the nation' (p. 133). Hegemony refers to the ongoing process whereby those in power manipulate public discourse (written and verbal), images and representations of people to benefit their own needs and maintain power. For example, in the past people with mental illnesses were portrayed in films such as *One Flew Over the Cuckoo's Nest* and *The Fisher King* as dangerous, crazy, mad, homicidal 'lunatics', people to be avoided at the very least, but more often feared and best 'managed' in asylums. Such portrayals of individuals with mental illnesses were also found in books, theatre, the media and other contributors to public discourse. So pervasive, insidious and persistent were these images over time that they created an everyday, common-sense understanding of mental illness regardless of the severity or type of mental health problems that people experienced.

The type of understanding described above exemplifies ideology, which Hammell (2006) defines as 'a system of ideas, beliefs and assumptions that operates below one's level of conscious awareness and, by being taken for granted, appears to constitute normal common sense' (p. 205). Thus, the creation and maintenance of seemingly self-evident truths and assumptions (ideology), for example people with mental health problems are dangerous and should be locked up, sustains unequal relations among groups within society while privileging those already in power (hegemony). When ideologies remain uncontested then society implicitly consents to, in this example, people with mental illnesses receiving unequal access to health care, employment, education, housing and social opportunities.

The ideology of independence, discussed in Chapter 1, represents another example of an ideology that remains relatively uncontested within rehabilitation professions, despite challenges from disability studies scholars and activists. Ideologies of professionalism have traditionally justified, legitimated and privileged professional knowledge and authority (Hammell, 2006). Rehabilitation professionals, with their ideology of "normality", their claim to "expert" status and their pretence of objectivity, are perceived to contribute to the oppression experienced by disabled people (French & Swain cited in Hammell, 2006, p. 149). The ongoing development of the client-centered model of practice represents rehabilitation professionals' attempts to challenge the status quo in health care. Qualitative research, in using an inductive and contextualized inquiry approach focused on research participants' accounts, is well suited to explore how ideologies privilege one group over another and influence disabled people's lives. Ideologies would appear to be inseparable from the theories and knowledge valued by professional groups that form the basis of the clinical reasoning process. It is, therefore, important that professionals understand the nature of their knowledge and how it is generated.

Professional knowledge and reasoning

Physical therapy and occupational therapy are pragmatic disciplines that draw on different types of knowledge and clinical reasoning to provide optimal intervention choices that can help clients resolve their problems. An understanding of the different approaches used in education and practice to generate knowledge and develop theory, such as deductive and inductive reasoning, helps to position qualitative research within specific knowledge traditions.

Deductive approaches to knowledge development start with the general, proposing a theory and testing a hypothesis, and end with explanations that aim to predict or establish causal relationships between phenomena. Quantitative research begins with an explicit theory already in place, 'and the research design evolves to test hypotheses concerning relevant relationships within the theory. This is a deductive line of reasoning where the rule or theory is stated and the examples or applications unfold in a way that fits the rule' (Ritchie, 2001, p. 151). The classic deductive literary figure is Sherlock Holmes, and his popular cultural counterpart is embodied in the television character 'Dr House' and his ability to make clinical diagnoses. In contrast, *inductive* approaches are a hallmark of qualitative research and are grounded in the social processes that people engage in and the meanings that they create from their experiences. Knowledge development using inductive approaches begins with the specific, observing particular people in context, and ends with descriptions and concepts that generate new social theories or contribute to and refine existing ones. In order to build a theory or conceptual model an inductive reasoning approach is taken. In this approach 'empirical observations are undertaken, providing data which, in turn, can be examined and categorized, leading to theory development' (Ritchie, 2001, p. 151). As LeCompte & Preissle (cited by Ritchie, 2001) state, 'in a sense, deductive researchers hope to find data to match a theory; inductive researchers hope to find a theory that explains their data' (p. 151).

Different forms of knowledge emanate from these two approaches and students use these to learn and practice their professions (Higgs *et al.*, 2001). Higgs & Titchen (1995) categorize knowledge as propositional or scientific, professional craft, and personal. *Propositional knowledge* is associated with causal factors, problem identification, diagnosis and generalizability (Higgs *et al.*, 2001). For example, practitioners draw on propositional knowledge to understand multiple sclerosis when they learn about the physiology of the deteriorating myelin sheath, recognize the presenting signs and symptoms, and predict diminishing function over time. *Professional craft or practice knowledge* combines previous general learning about disability or a health condition, or situation and a client's unique experience, within a particular context. Thus, practitioners anticipate the physical functioning of a person with multiple sclerosis but may also explore issues such as housing, social support, income, physical surroundings and psychological response to develop a holistic understanding of the specific individual's experience of the condition. Lastly, *personal knowledge* arises from a tacit understanding of the practitioner's life experiences and also, ideally, from a conscious self-reflection on previous therapeutic encounters. Socialization to professional values such as treating clients with respect, recognizing their inherent worth and dignity, and working collaboratively all contribute to the development of personal knowledge.

Basic scientific knowledge is needed in rehabilitation, but there has been an over-reliance on this approach (Forsyth *et al.*, 2005). The limited use of theory by occupational therapists and physical therapists in the UK (see Roskell *et al.*, 1998; Forsyth *et al.*, 2005) and the United States (see De Souza, 1998; Elliot *et al.*, 2002) can be traced, in part, to 'knowledge production based on "technical rationality", the idea that practical action flows naturally from basic knowledge' (Forsyth *et al.*, 2005, p. 261). This has distracted rehabilitation professionals from developing theories that could illuminate crucial problems and issues associated with the illness experience and impairment. Physical therapists and occupational therapists would be more likely to draw on theories to guide practice if those theories were grounded in the multi-layered social, cultural, economic and physical experiences that comprise their clients' lives. Nixon & Creek's (2006) call for theorizing within everyday occupational therapy practice alludes to the potential of qualitative research. They write:

> We *do* theory by developing collaborative models of thoughtful practice that challenge assumptions and suggest new lines of inquiry; we *do* theory by learning how to align thoughtfulness and practice within specific contexts that require constant negotiation across complex professional, cultural and social boundaries (p. 81).

The practices of collaborating, contesting assumptions and attending to contexts are found within the philosophical perspectives that contribute to qualitative research and that continue to shape it. These practices reflect interdisciplinary post-modern thinking and contrast sharply with positivist inquiry approaches to knowledge development.

Characteristics of qualitative research

Qualitative research is inductive

An inductive approach to knowledge generation is a key characteristic of qualitative research. This approach is grounded in observations of day-to-day life and aims to establish linkages between social phenomena or inferences about situations. It is used to bring knowledge into view, and to develop theories and create concepts. Thus, researchers generate data from various sources (research participants, key informants, family members, service providers) and use methods such as participant observation, in-depth interviewing, document analysis and life history. Health policy researchers Murphy & Dingwall (2003) reject the assumption that qualitative research is 100% inductive. They suggest instead that researchers tend either to emphasize theoretical development that borders on hypothesis testing or focus more closely on data generation. The methodological choice a researcher makes also influences the extent to which induction is used in more deductive approaches, for example grounded theory is located closer to the deduction end of the knowledge generation continuum than is phenomenology.

Qualitative research is interpretive

The interpretive nature of qualitative research is one of its defining characteristics and informs the participant's point of view, the role of the researcher, the context of the study and the presentation of findings. The participant's point of view or interpretation reflects their subjective state; a conglomeration of emotions, perceptions and intentions that are only known to that individual. Subjectivity is not merely one's conscious thought, but includes 'the role played by social relations and language in determining, regulating and producing what a "thinking subject" can be' (O'Sullivan, 1994, p. 309). An aim of qualitative inquiry is to understand and explore the concept of *intersubjectivity* that we briefly discussed in Chapter 1. Intersubjectivity is 'a social accomplishment, a set of understandings sustained in and through the shared assumptions of interactions' (Gubrium & Holstein, 2000, p. 489). It forms the background against which individuals struggle to make sense of problems and unsettling situations. Through intersubjectivity everyday life is interpreted in typical ways within a framework of familiarity. It occurs when subjectivity is expressed through language, as happens during interviews, when the researcher is able to take the position of the research participant (Carspecken, 1996). Qualitative research seeks to understand and reflect the *emic* or insider's point of view, that is, the perspective of the individual or group who has lived through and interpreted an experience or ongoing circumstances. The experiential aspect of phenomena is valued even though it may differ from objective accounts of what occurred or what rehabilitation professionals deem to be important. The concept of multiple realities, which can broaden professional knowledge, is explored further as it relates to qualitative research as an interpretive endeavor.

Multiple realities

A key characteristic of qualitative research is that there are multiple realities or truths that can be understood by exploring the meanings that people ascribe to their experiences and interactions in the social world. The notion of multiple realities draws heavily from constructivism and refers to the different and yet 'valid' interpretations that people have about their lives and the social structures that shape their lives. The experience of growing up in a family provides an example of multiple realities. Most families would agree about objective information such as where the family had lived, what their income and employment status was, and when major events such as births, deaths and coming of age ceremonies occurred. Each family member is likely, however, to have a unique interpretation of these experiences and could create a narrative that is at odds with that of another family member. The Personal Narratives Group (1989) captured the idea of multiple realities in discussing how people interpret their lives:

> When talking about their lives, people lie sometimes, forget a lot, exaggerate, become confused, and get things wrong. Yet they *are* revealing truths. These truths don't reveal the past 'as it actually was', aspiring to a standard of objectivity. They give us instead the truths of our experiences. They aren't the result of empirical research or the logic of mathematical deductions. Unlike the reassuring Truth of the scientific ideal, the truths of personal narratives are neither open to proof nor self-evident. We come to understand them only through interpretation, paying careful attention to the contexts that shape their creation and the worldviews that inform them (p. 261).

Laliberte-Rudman *et al.* (2006) sought out the perspectives of people who used wheelchairs after a cerebral vascular accident in order to understand how this life change shaped their occupational lives. Although the finding that multiple physical environmental barriers exist could have been anticipated, the losses related to leisure and social activities that participants described offer rehabilitation professionals a unique insider view of life post-stroke and have implications for community-based practice. The extent to which most researchers, who are typically positioned as outsiders with an *etic* perspective, can produce an emic account is debatable, but the incorporation and valuing of insiders' voices in knowledge development is clearly increasing within the rehabilitation professions.

Researcher as research instrument

The active role that the qualitative researcher plays in producing findings that contribute to knowledge development differs from the role a researcher takes within positivist methodologies. The constructivist idea of knowledge as a joint endeavor rather than a lone discovery of truth, and the recognition that research participants and the researcher interact in a shared social world (to a greater or lesser extent), position the researcher as 'his or her own research instrument' (Punch, 1994, p. 84). This statement refers to the involvement that researchers have in negotiating meanings, the impact they have on the data generation process and the relationship they form with research participants. To ensure that the findings are authentic and credible, researchers must examine and come to understand how their position in the social world influences the study, that is, they must engage in reflexivity. This topic will be addressed more fully in Chapter 7.

Setting and context

Another characteristic of qualitative research, which has its roots in cultural anthropology and sociology, is the value placed on studying social processes and how people make sense of themselves within particular contexts (Denzin & Lincoln, 2005). There is a tradition of anthropologists living in foreign cultures and studying the everyday practices and activities of the people, and in doing so, gaining an understanding of a culture and its members. Thus, the credibility of the data relies on its being contextualized, that is, described and explained within a particular place and time in history. *Context* is a critical framework for learning how people with chronic health conditions and disabled people live outside hospitals and institutions. Most qualitative researchers strive to conduct their studies in settings or contexts that are naturalistic, that is, the environments in which the phenomena of interest typically occur. If, for example, rehabilitation professionals want to understand which skills and strategies are most relevant to their clients' lives, the researchers would want to locate the research and generate data in clients' day-to-day environments of community, home, school and/or work. Primeau's (2003) research in the homes of families highlights the importance of studying a phenomenon in the most natural setting possible and the inseparability of data from the contexts in which they arise.

Physical therapy and occupational therapy researchers can learn about their respective professional cultures by studying practice settings, which may reveal implicit beliefs and attitudes that underpin their expectations of clients and the therapy that is subsequently offered. Richardson (2006) describes how direct observation provided insights into the ways in which physical therapists apply knowledge to practice. Through the use of video observations and on-site interviews Richardson built a different understanding of physical therapy culture to what would have been possible by using, for example, questionnaires or reflective diaries as data collection methods. She created an in-depth description of processes that occurred in three diverse physical therapy practice settings and incorporated these findings into her practice as an educator.

Descriptive nature of data

A key characteristic of qualitative research is the highly descriptive form that the data take and the presentation of findings that typically include verbatim quotations from participants that illustrate and substantiate the analysis. The detailed narrative forms that a researcher creates from interviews, observations, videotapes, public and private documents, analytic memos, field notes and other data aims to preserve the participants' words and style of expression. Qualitative research is concerned with the interpretation of meanings, contexts and processes and this requires a particular style of report or writing. Holloway (2005) proposes that 'the reader of a piece of qualitative research should be able to reconstruct a vivid picture of the world of the participants, therefore the research report must grip the reader's attention and imagination, and tell a compelling story' (p. 270). Descriptive writing and quotations from participants are central to painting a vivid picture that answers the research question.

Interaction between participant and researcher

Extensive interaction between the researcher and the participants is another characteristic of good qualitative inquiry (Avis, 2005). This type of interaction may comprise a series of in-depth interviews or many hours of observation and participation in the contexts of interest over weeks and months. The latter interactions may be unstructured, as is sometimes the case with participant observation. The aim of extensive interaction is to allow the researcher to take part in the social world of the participants, to varying degrees, and to enhance the credibility of the data. This approach positions the researcher as a student or a learner, someone who is interested in understanding participants' perspectives and the meanings that they create based on how they perceive their circumstances. Lastly, the extent and duration of interaction with participants may prompt researchers to refine or change the focus of inquiry as the study progresses.

Flexible nature of the research design

Flexibility of the research design during the study is characteristic of qualitative inquiry and is consistent with the aim of exploring and describing phenomena (Bogdan & Biklen, 2003). Despite having reviewed the literature on a topic or phenomenon (assuming literature exists), researchers do not necessarily know which questions are important to pursue until they have spent time in the setting and/or talked to people who experience the situation. Although thesis committees and ethical review boards require a precise and well-designed research question, we agree with Bogdan & Biklen (2003), who advocate having a general question in mind and then entering the *field* or setting to watch, listen and learn. Thus, a researcher engages in a sort of reconnaissance mission, and through initial data generation works inductively toward a clear articulation of the research question and the suitable data gathering methods. This inductive approach results in a less linear research design than is typical or appropriate for a quantitative methodology.

Nature of qualitative data

Qualitative data can be derived from interaction with participants, such as interviews or focus groups, or as a result of participant observation or analysis of documents or records. Qualitative data, whether in the form of transcripts or field notes, are generally presented in narrative form. When derived from inter-action with participants the data are presented as verbatim quotations, to pre-serve and represent the *voices* of the participants. In addition to generating an in-depth, descriptive *narrative* of the participants' accounts, qualitative data also take the form of descriptions or stories that represent interpretations made by the researcher for the purpose of enabling readers to have a better understanding of particular people and circumstances. To define qualitative research as merely stories, however, provides a partial definition and one that is insufficient for know-ledge development in occupational therapy and physical therapy. Well-designed qualitative research can generate new understanding and conceptual knowledge and contribute to developing and refining theories that are relevant to client service provision.

Linking theory to practice

'Theory, although understated (or even unstated), is what guides all clinical prac-tice and every research inquiry: informing what practitioners believe should be done in various situations' (Hammell & Carpenter, 2000, p. 10). Important devel-opments in rehabilitation, such as evidence-based and client-centered models of practice, have revealed what has been called the theory–practice gap. This gap is illustrated by the divergence of holistic and biomechanical approaches to rehab-ilitation therapy, perceived inconsistencies between professional education and clinical practice, and the gap between the 'best' research evidence and the reality of practice (Roskell *et al.*, 1998). 'The role of theory in guiding clinical practice and research inquiry, and thus informing how rehabilitation professionals respond to individual client circumstances, has rarely been made explicit' (Carpenter, 2004a, p. 8). It has become an imperative that the theories, concepts and assumptions central to rehabilitation practice be systematically examined. Client-centered practice, neuro-developmental approaches to treatment, leisure and spirituality are examples of under-researched theoretical concepts in physical therapy and occu-pational therapy. Qualitative research can be used 'to surface hidden theoretical assumptions and suggest new possibilities and connections' (Miller & Crabtree, 2005, p. 618). Rebeiro & Cook's (1999) study of occupation as a means to mental health exemplifies this potential. Their exploratory study focused on the belief that occupation, a theoretical concept supported in the literature but lacking empirical research, enhances mental health. The focus of their study was an out-patient women's group where Rebeiro (as principal investigator) used occupation as a sensitizing concept after observing that occupation seemed to differentiate this group from other mental health groups. Rebeiro & Cook (1999) developed a conceptual model from the findings that described how members experienced the group (affirming), how this led to increased feelings of esteem (confirming), and how these stages facilitated a process of occupational engagement (occupational spin-off). These findings served program evaluation needs and illustrated the significance of the social environment in encouraging occupational engagement, and thus furthered the theoretical development of occupation.

Rehabilitation, as Hammell (2006) suggests, 'is more than a physical endeavor. It is not about treating and curing, but about living' (p. 107). The therapeutic or healing process does not only occur in the rehabilitation context but also in everyday life. However, the theoretical basis of rehabilitation has been largely generated without client input and this absence of clients' perspectives provides an unstable basis from which to inform client-centered rehabilitation practice (Hammell, 2004). Qualitative research offers the opportunity to study how clients apply and make meaning of rehabilitation interventions in their everyday lives. In the remainder of this chapter we will discuss how qualitative research can inform contemporary rehabilitation practice.

The contribution of qualitative research to contemporary rehabilitation practice

Evidence-based practice

The rehabilitation disciplines have willingly subscribed to the evidence-based practice movement and its culture of accountability (Carpenter, 2004a). The concept of evidence-based practice evolved from a problem-based learning strategy developed for medical education at McMaster University, Canada, in 1992. Sackett *et al.* (2000) further defined the concept as 'the integration of best research evidence with clinical expertise and patient values' (p. 1). This definition clearly acknowledges the important role of clinical experience, clinical wisdom and intuition in making use of the 'best' evidence in meeting 'the unique preferences, concerns and expectations each patient brings to the clinical encounter' (Sackett *et al.*, 2000, p. 1).

Primary criticisms of evidence-based practice have been based on the perception that evidence derived from experimental research has been privileged, that such evidence is neither relevant nor applicable to complex clinical situations and contexts, that clinical expertise is undervalued, and that patients' perspectives are rarely taken into account. Many of these criticisms have been addressed as rehabilitation therapists assumed the responsibility of accountability, adopted an analytical approach to practice and developed the skills needed to access evidence. Effective integration of evidence-based practice is dependent on rehabilitation therapists developing their clinical expertise, knowledge and judgment. Qualitative research can contribute to an understanding of the nature of clinical reasoning and how professional knowledge is developed and transmitted. Gwyer *et al.* (2004) describe how they used a multiple qualitative case-study research approach to develop an understanding of clinical expertise. Their findings reflect the scope of evidence needed to address clients' goals in a relevant and effective manner and provide evidence to support the development of physical therapy theory and educational strategies that promote evidence-based practice in rehabilitation (Carpenter, 2004a).

Another concern, identified by rehabilitation therapists, is the perceived constraining nature of the standardized outcome measures available for use in rehabilitation. Many outcome measures lack the sensitivity needed to capture a client's functional level or improvement, particularly given the decreased client admission times and lack of formal follow-up services. Rehabilitation interventions are designed with the client's larger context and goals in mind and in collaboration with other members of the interdisciplinary team. Establishing the efficacy of interventions is less important than ensuring the effectiveness, that is, that interventions are based on the best available evidence and applied within real-life conditions. The focus on the use of outcomes and ensuring effectiveness informs the choices of health professionals and organizations, provides accountability and improves care from a management perspective, but leaves many voices, particularly the clients', unheard and questions unanswered (Miller & Crabtree, 2005). Qualitative research can contribute to the development and evaluation of outcome measures that reflect the clients' goals and priorities, for example the Canadian Occupational Performance Measure (COPM) (Law *et al.*, 2005). More importantly, qualitative research approaches are ideally suited to explore clients' health beliefs and related experiences, and their perceptions of the therapeutic relationship and the complexities of rehabilitation practice. Cooper *et al.* (2005) conducted a study to elicit patients' beliefs about the role of cardiac rehabilitation following myocardial infarction. The findings clearly identified the need to address the misconceptions that patients and their relatives may have regarding coronary heart disease more explicitly. Blank (2004) sought to explore the experience of working in partnership with occupational therapists in community mental health from the client's perspective. Interestingly, the personality and behavior of the therapist emerged as being of primary importance to the clients.

One of the central assumptions of qualitative research, as described earlier, is the need to understand the context within which the experience or situation occurs. In order to provide evidence of effective intervention or service, the clients' everyday context needs to be considered. Heckman & Cott (2005) demonstrated how a qualitative approach could be used to achieve a better understanding of the practice of physical therapy within the context of the elderly clients' home. Beardwood *et al.* (2005) described the qualitative component of a larger participatory action research project involving injured workers that aimed to understand their injury experiences in the context of insufficient compensation and inability to return to satisfactory employment. Such research exemplifies the contribution that participants who are service users can make in constructing unique evidence and developing theory that is grounded in people's experiences and their own settings.

Client-centered practice

Client-centered practice in rehabilitation has been defined as a collaborative approach to service 'whereby clients engage the assistance and support of a therapist to facilitate their problem solving and the achievement of their own goals' (McColl *et al.* cited in Hammell & Carpenter, 2004, p. 7). Client-centered therapists 'demonstrate respect for clients, involve clients in decision-making, advocate with and for clients in meeting clients' needs, and otherwise recognize clients' experience and knowledge' (Canadian Association of Occupational Therapists cited by Law, 1998, p. 3). Occupational therapy has taken a leading role in developing the theoretical concept of client-centered practice as evidenced in numerous articles, texts and guides (for example Law, 1998; Corring & Cook, 1999; Sumsion, 1999). Although physical therapists claim to be engaged in client/patient-centered practice, professional publications on this topic are scarce (Carpenter, 2004b). Townsend *et al.* (2003) describe how an institutional ethnographic approach to research contributed to understanding and transforming the professional tensions in client-centered practice. They recognized that in reality:

> Client-centered practice is fraught with tensions. Notable struggles in trying to be client-centered are embedded in finding time to work collaboratively with people, and in stretching services to work with the whole person, their environment, and their overall occupational [or functional] performance' (p. 18).

Hammell (2006) suggests that client-centered practice 'should be regarded as a goal rather than a reality, with changes in rehabilitation practice lagging behind changes in political and professional rhetoric' (p. 154). As yet, there is insufficient research that explores the meaning of client-centered practice or evaluates how it is provided in the real world of clinical practice. Corring (2004) provides an example in her description of a participatory action research approach that involved users of mental health services. The aim of the research was to explore how the participants define client-centered care and their quality of life issues, with the purpose of ensuring a client perspective in the development of evidence-based mental health services.

Assessing quality of life

Despite the lack of consensus on a definition, there is a great emphasis on quality of life as an overall goal of rehabilitation. As we discussed in Chapter 1, there is a plethora of literature describing attempts to define quality of life, to measure it, research it and incorporate data from assessments into policy decisions, and yet the interest in examining the assumptions underlying the concept has been primarily from disability scholars and activists (Priestly, 2003). Hammell (2006) argues that the 'optimal client outcomes' identified in evidence-based articles are more likely based on therapists' values and definitions of a quality life than those of the client (p. 137). Laliberte-Rudman *et al.* (2000) explored the perspectives of people with schizophrenia regarding the meaning of quality of life and factors perceived to be important to quality of life. Although their findings corroborated the factors usually included in quality of life assessments, the participants provided new insights and priorities about what was important to them. This type of qualitative evidence supports the development of meaningful and relevant rehabilitation services for people living with chronic conditions or disability.

Qualitative research conducted in conjunction with other research approaches

Qualitative methodologies can be combined with quantitative or survey methodologies using a mixed method approach and these are discussed in more detail in Chapter 10. Qualitative research can provide theoretical explanations for the results of quantitative studies that are usually expressed in terms of relations between variables. It can shed light on the complex processes, such as adherence, or self-management of a therapeutic regimen, or motivation to follow exercise recommendations, that are not captured by conducting a quantitative study (Grypdonck, 2006). Quantitative studies focus on cause and effect relations and on routine standardized procedures. 'Qualitative understanding, and especially qualitative theory construction, can contribute to the awareness of the practitioner of the factors that are important in a situation that require adaptation of the routine procedure' (Grypdonck, 2006, p. 1380) and enable experimental research findings to be contextualized.

In summary, in this chapter we have argued that qualitative research can contribute substantially and in different ways to rehabilitation practice by challenging taken-for-granted practices; illuminating factors that shape client and professional behaviors; developing new interventions based on clients' experiences; evaluating and determining optimal outcomes of care; enhancing understanding of organizational culture and the management of change; and evaluating service delivery. In the next chapter, we will draw on the issues discussed in the previous two chapters, and provide an overview of the components of the research planning process and discuss how they can be integrated effectively to develop a research study proposal or submit an ethics approval application.

References

Avis, M. (2005) Is there an epistemology for qualitative research? In: I. Holloway (ed.), *Qualitative Research in Health Care* (pp. 3–16). Oxford, Open University Press.

Backman, C.L., Del-Fabro Smith, L., Smith, S., Montie, P.L. & Suto, M. (2007) The experiences of mothers living with inflammatory arthritis. *Arthritis and Rheumatism (Arthritis Care & Research)*, 57, 381–388.

Beardwood, B.A., Kirsh, B. & Clark, N.J. (2005) Victims twice over: perceptions and experiences of injured workers. *Qualitative Health Research*, 15 (1), 30–48.

Blank, A. (2004) Clients' experiences of partnership with occupational therapists in community mental health. *British Journal of Occupational Therapy*, 67 (3), 118–124.

Bogdan, R.C. & Biklen, S.K. (2003) *Qualitative Research for Education: an Introduction to Theory and Methods* (4th edn). Boston, Allyn & Bacon.

Carpenter, C. (2004a) The contribution of qualitative research to evidence-based practice. In: K.W. Hammell & C. Carpenter (eds), *Qualitative Research in Evidence-based Rehabilitation* (pp. 1–13). Edinburgh, Churchill Livingstone.

Carspecken, P.F. (1996) *Critical Ethnography in Educational Research: a Theoretical and Practical Guide*. New York, Routledge.

Carpenter, C. (2004b) Dilemmas of practice as experienced by physical therapists in rehabilitation settings. *Physiotherapy Canada*, 57 (1), 63–74.

Cooper, A.F., Jackson, G., Weinman, J. & Horne, R. (2005) A qualitative study investigating patients' beliefs about cardiac rehabilitation. *Clinical Rehabilitation*, 19, 87–96.

Corring, D. (2004) Ensuring a client perspective in evidence-based rehabilitation research. In: K.W. Hammell & C. Carpenter (eds), *Qualitative Research in Evidence-based Rehabilitation* (pp. 65–76). Edinburgh, Churchill Livingstone.

Corring, D. & Cook, J.V. (1999) Client-centered care means that I am a valued human being. *Canadian Journal of Occupational Therapy*, 66 (2), 71–82.

Crepeau, E.B., Cohn, E.S. & Boyt Schell, B.A. (2003) *Willard and Spackman's Occupational Therapy* (10th edn). Philadelphia, Lippincott Williams & Wilkins.

Creswell, J., Hanson, W.E., Clark, V.L.P. & Morales, A. (2007) Qualitative research designs: selection and implementation. *The Counselling Psychologist*, 35 (2), 236–264.

Denzin, N.K. & Lincoln, Y.S. (2005) Introduction: the discipline and practice of qualitative research. In: N.K. Denzin & Y.S. Lincoln (eds), *The Sage Handbook of Qualitative Research* (3rd edn, pp. 1–32). Thousand Oaks, Calif., Sage.

De Souza, L. (1998) Editorial – theories about therapies are underdeveloped. *Physiotherapy Research International*, 3 (3), iv–vi.

Dyson, S. & Brown, B. (2006) *Social Theory and Applied Health Research*. Oxford, Open University Press.

Elliot, S.J., Velde, B.P. & Wittman, P.P. (2002) The use of theory in everyday practice: an exploratory study. *Occupational Therapy in Health Care*, 16 (1), 45–62.

Forsyth, K., Summerfield Mann, L. & Kielhofner, G. (2005) Scholarship of practice: making occupation-focused, theory-driven, evidence-based practice a reality. *British Journal of Occupational Therapy*, 68 (6), 260–268.

Grypdonck, M.H.F. (2006) Qualitative health research in the era of evidence-based practice. *Qualitative Health Research*, 16 (10), 1371–1385.

Guba, E.G. & Lincoln, Y.S. (2005) Paradigmatic controversies, contradictions, and emerging confluences. In: N.K. Denzin & Y.S. Lincoln (eds), *The Sage Handbook of Qualitative Research* (3rd edn, pp. 191–215). Thousand Oaks, Calif., Sage.

Gubrium, J. & Holstein, J. (2000) Analyzing interpretive practice. In: N. Denzin & Y. Lincoln (eds), *Handbook of Qualitative Research* (2nd edn, pp. 487–508). Thousand Oaks, Calif., Sage.

Gwyer, J., Jensen, G., Hack, L. & Shepard, K. (2004) Using a multiple case-study research design to develop an understanding of clinical expertise in physical therapy. In: K.W. Hammell & C. Carpenter (eds), *Qualitative Research in Evidence-based Rehabilitation* (pp. 103–115). Edinburgh, Churchill Livingstone.

Hammell, K.W. (2004) Quality of life among people with high spinal cord injury living in the community. *Spinal Cord*, 42 (11), 607–620.

Hammell, K.W. (2006) *Perspectives on Disability and Rehabilitation: Contesting Assumptions, Challenging Practice*. Edinburgh, Churchill Livingstone/Elsevier.

Hammell, K.W. & Carpenter, C. (2000) Introduction to qualitative research in occupational therapy and physical therapy. In: K.W. Hammell, C. Carpenter & I. Dyck (eds), *Using Qualitative Research: a Practical Introduction for Occupational and Physical Therapists* (pp. 1–12). Edinburgh, Churchill Livingstone.

Hammell, K.W. & Carpenter, C. (2004) *Qualitative Research in Evidence-based Rehabilitation*. Edinburgh, Churchill Livingstone.

Heckman, K.A. & Cott, C.A. (2005) Home-based physiotherapy for the elderly: a different world. *Physiotherapy Canada*, 57, 274–283.

Higgs, J. & Titchen, A. (1995) Propositional, professional and personal knowledge in clinical reasoning. In: J. Higgs & M. Jones (eds), *Clinical Reasoning in the Health Professions* (pp. 129–146). Oxford, Butterworth-Heinemann.

Higgs, J., Titchen, A. & Neville, V. (2001) Professional practice and knowledge. In: J. Higgs & A. Titchen (eds), *Practice Knowledge and Expertise* (pp. 3–9). Oxford, Butterworth-Heinemann.

Holloway, I. (2005) Qualitative writing. In: I. Holloway (ed.), *Qualitative Research in Health Care* (pp. 270–286). Oxford, Open University Press.

Kincheloe, J.L. & McLaren, P. (2005) Rethinking critical theory and qualitative research. In: N.K. Denzin & Y.S. Lincoln (eds), *The Sage Handbook of Qualitative Research* (3rd edn, pp. 303–342). Thousand Oaks, Calif., Sage.

Laliberte-Rudman, D., Yu, B., Scott, E. & Pajouhandeh, P. (2000) Exploration of the perspectives of persons with schizophrenia regarding quality of life. *American Journal of Occupational Therapy*, 54 (2), 137–147.

Laliberte-Rudman, D., Hebert, D. & Reid, D. (2006) Living in a restricted occupational world: the occupational experiences of stroke survivors who are wheelchair users and their caregivers. *Canadian Journal of Occupational Therapy*, 73 (3), 141–152.

Lather, P. (1991) *Getting Smart: Feminist Research and Pedagogy with/in the Postmodern*. New York, Routledge.

Law, M. (ed.) (1998) *Client-centered Occupational Therapy*. Thorofare, NJ, Slack.

Law, M., Baptiste, S., McColl, M., Opzoomer, A., Pollock, N. & Polatajko, H. (2005) *Canadian Occupational Performance Measure*. Retrieved 3 March 2007 from: http://www.caot.ca/copm/index.htm

Miller, W.L. & Crabtree, B.F. (2005) Clinical research. In: N.K. Denzin & Y.S. Lincoln (eds), *The Sage Handbook of Qualitative Research* (pp. 605–639). Thousand Oaks, Calif., Sage.

Murphy, E. & Dingwall, R. (2003) *Qualitative Methods and Health Policy Research*. New York, Aldine De Gruyter.

Nixon, J. & Creek, J. (2006) Towards a theory of practice. *British Journal of Occupational Therapy*, 69, 77–80.

O'Sullivan, T., Hartley, J., Saunders, D. & Montgomery, M. (1994) *Key Concepts in Communication and Cultural Studies*. London, Routledge.

Personal Narratives Group (1989) Truths. In: Personal Narratives Group (eds), *Interpreting Women's Lives: Feminist Theory and Personal Narratives* (pp. 261–264). Bloomington, Ind., Indiana University Press.

Priestly, M. (2003) *Disability: a Life Course Approach*. Cambridge, Polity.

Primeau, L.A. (2003) Reflections on self in qualitative research: stories of family. *American Journal of Occupational Therapy*, 57 (1), 9–16.

Punch, M. (1994) Politics and ethics in qualitative research. In: N.K. Denzin & Y.S. Lincoln (eds), *Handbook of Qualitative Research* (pp. 83–97). Thousand Oaks, Calif., Sage.

Rapport, F. (2005) Hermeneutic phenomenology: the science of interpretation of texts. In: I. Holloway (ed.), *Qualitative Research in Health Care* (pp. 125–146). Oxford, Open University Press.

Rebeiro, K. & Cook, J.V. (1999) Opportunity, not prescription: an exploratory study of the experience of occupational engagement. *Canadian Journal of Occupational Therapy*, 66 (4), 176–187.

Richardson, B. (2006) An ethnography of physiotherapy culture. In: L. Finlay & C. Ballinger (eds), *Qualitative Research for Allied Health Professional: Challenging Choices* (pp. 79–92). Chichester, UK, Whurr Publications.

Ritchie, J. (2001) Not everything can be reduced to numbers. In: C. Berglund (ed.), *Health Research* (pp. 149–271). Oxford, Oxford University Press.

Roskell, C., Hewison, A. & Wildman, S. (1998) The theory–practice gap and physiotherapy in the UK: insights from the nursing experience. *Physiotherapy Theory and Practice*, 14, 223–233.

Sackett, D.L., Strauss, S.E., Richardson, W.S., Rosenberg, W. & Haynes, R.B. (2000) *Evidence-based Medicine: How to Practice and Teach EBP* (2nd edn). Edinburgh, Churchill Livingstone.

Sakellariou, D. & Algado, S.S. (2006) Sexuality and disability: a case of occupational injustice. *British Journal of Occupational Therapy*, 69 (2), 69–76.

Schutz, A. (1970) *On Phenomenology and Social Relations; Selected Writings*. H.R. Wagner (ed.). Chicago, The University of Chicago Press.

Schwandt, T. (2000) Three epistemological stances for qualitative inquiry: interpretivism, hermeneutics and social constructivism. In: N. Denzin & Y. Lincoln (eds), *Handbook of Qualitative Research* (2nd edn, pp. 189–214). Thousand Oaks, Calif., Sage.

Sumsion, T. (ed.) (1999) *Client-centered Practice in Occupational Therapy: a Guide to Implementation*. Edinburgh, Churchill Livingstone.

Townsend, E., Langille, L. & Ripley, D. (2003) Professional tensions in client-centered practice: using institutional ethnography to generate understanding and transformation. *American Journal of Occupational Therapy*, 57 (1), 17–28.

Chapter 3
DEVELOPING A RESEARCH PLAN

Introduction

In this chapter, we provide an overview of the research design process by describing and justifying the different decisions that need to be made in developing a qualitative research project. In our experience, some people learn by acquiring a sense of the whole picture and then exploring the components in detail, whilst others prefer to build upon the component parts. This chapter represents the whole picture and our purpose is to introduce each component and explore how they are linked to form a logical and integrated approach to the proposed research. This type of approach is also required in writing a qualitative research proposal for seeking either ethical approval, funding or agency sponsorship. The emergent nature of qualitative research requires a flexible approach, but this does not exempt the researcher from making a comprehensive and balanced argument for the study design. In reality, the design may require modification of the research question at a later stage because interaction with participants may present the phenomena or problem differently from how the researcher originally thought, but a rigorous and well-conceived initial plan is essential.

An effective research design includes establishing the research purpose and developing the research question, conducting a literature review, choosing an appropriate qualitative methodology and data collection method, recruiting participants and determining the data analysis approach. Throughout the design process, careful consideration must be paid to the role of the researcher and the ethical issues inherent in conducting qualitative research. These design components will each be discussed in detail in subsequent chapters.

There are many potential research questions but our interest lies in focusing on the ones that, when answered, will make some difference to clients' lives and educate rehabilitation professionals. We think it is essential that researchers take the time during this process to become aware of the implicit assumptions, gained through professional education and practice, that shape how they think about illness, disability and health, and subsequently, what kinds of questions they will articulate. In this chapter we also address the practicalities of planning a research project, such as managing the data, outlining a timeline and developing a budget.

Establishing the research purpose

The overall purpose of qualitative research can be broadly described as descriptive, exploratory, explanatory or emancipatory. *Descriptive research*, as its name suggests, provides a rich descriptive account of a phenomenon within a context and an established framework of knowledge. It is likely that, as a result of studying the existing literature, the fundamental concepts related to the topic will already have been identified (Sim & Wright, 2000). However, in this type of research, the aim will be to 'produce a fuller account of the phenomenon and perhaps quantify some of the key concepts or variables', and in addition, 'the researcher will probably wish to identify some relationships of potential theoretical interest' (Sim & Wright, 2000, p. 19). Ethnographic researchers often invoke Geertz's (1973) concept of *thick description* to convey the depth of portrayal entailed in this type of research. The purpose of thick description may also be to develop in more detail an established theory or body of knowledge. A descriptive purpose can also entail developing systematic lists of concepts or topics that are similar, ordered or related, for example using a consensus technique (Delphi or nominal group) to rank priorities, develop a taxonomy of illness terms used by a group, or to determine frequency of word use (see Chapter 5).

Exploratory research refers to inquiry that breaks new ground by examining experiences, situations and meanings and, in doing so, identifies concepts previously ignored or under-theorized in rehabilitation. Exploratory questions are typically broad, and researchers are motivated by a desire to find out more about what is happening, to seek new insights, or to assess phenomena from a new perspective. Exploratory research, in particular, reflects the emergent and flexible characteristic of qualitative research. Exploratory qualitative studies often focus on the experiences of people whose perspectives have not been represented in more traditional research. These may be individuals whose situations and diagnoses put them at the margins of mainstream health research, where their voices are unlikely to be heard (Corring & Cook, 1999; Hammell, 2004).

The purpose of *explanatory research* tends to be more specific than the preceding types of research, and is most often associated with quantitative research where the purpose is to test a hypothesis (Sim & Wright, 2000). However, some qualitative research projects can be described as having an explanatory rather than a descriptive purpose. In rehabilitation practice, explanatory research may focus on certain types of settings that form small cultural units such as Richardson's (2006) ethnographic study of how professional knowledge is integrated into physiotherapy practice. Other explanatory qualitative research aims to illuminate social processes specifically to create theoretical frameworks for further empirical research, as in the case of studies using a grounded theory approach.

Lastly, *emancipatory research* may have explanatory and descriptive elements but its primary aim is to facilitate change in people's lives and in their particular circumstances through the research process. Emancipatory research is associated with advocates of critical theories (see Chapter 2) who critique forms of power. The emancipatory research agenda acknowledges that research is a political process and is characterized by a number of core principles: control, accountability, empowerment, respect and collaboration. These principles are integral to participatory action research and this approach is discussed in more detail in Chapter 4.

Developing the research question

Qualitative research questions do not exist in a vacuum; they arise from somewhere and the genesis of inquiry for most physical therapists and occupational therapists is in practice. *Foreshadowed problems* or *clinical irritations* occur as practitioners reflect on client experiences that are puzzling, dissatisfying or intellectually confusing. The term 'foreshadowed problem' refers to viewing phenomena of interest (behavioral patterns, social processes) through particular theoretical lenses (Hammersley & Atkinson, 1995). For example, as an occupational therapist, Suto (2000) recognized that many people with chronic schizophrenia had difficulty structuring their time in ways that enabled meaningful occupations and she incorporated theories from psychology, sociology and occupational therapy in her efforts to explain her clinical observations. Carpenter (2000), as a physiotherapist coordinating a large research project, had the opportunity to talk with people who had been living in the community for many years after sustaining a spinal cord injury. These conversations reinforced her perception that there was a discrepancy between rehabilitation professionals' view of what living with a spinal cord injury would be like and the actual reality experienced by disabled people. In developing a conceptual framework for her research, Carpenter drew on the theoretical concepts of significant life events from psychology and transformational learning in adult education.

Research questions must be viewed within a particular theoretical context. A clinical irritation reveals certain theoretical concerns on the part of the researcher and may arise when some aspect of practice is puzzling and the literature, if there is any available, offers explanations that conflict with their experience or the clients'. *Sensitizing concepts* are the concepts that interest a researcher and develop from reflection-on-practice, discipline-specific concerns and one's worldview (Brown, 2006). Examples of sensitizing concepts include independence, adaptation, illness narratives, social class, cultural differences and biographical disruption. Sensitizing concepts are used to shape the early research phase and may later guide data analysis. The sensitizing concepts and theories that initially help to articulate the problem represent the researcher's conceptual framework. As Miles & Huberman (1994) explain: 'A conceptual framework explains, either graphically or in narrative form, the main things to be studied – the key factors, constructs or variables – and the [possible] relationships between them. Frameworks can be rudimentary, elaborate, theory-driven or commonsensical, descriptive or causal' (p. 18). It is important that researchers make their conceptual frameworks as explicit as possible because whether implicit, emerging or explicit, they will affect how the research question is articulated.

The type of research question informs the type of research, choice of qualitative methodology and methods of data collection. As Creswell *et al.* (2007) note: 'The old adage that the methods should be based on the research questions is seldom explained for investigators, especially those new to qualitative research' (p. 238). In our experience, novice researchers all too often begin by choosing a particular method, for example focus groups, and try to fit the research question to this choice. This approach fails to support the logic and credibility of a qualitative research design. Qualitative research questions are typically open-ended and act as a guide to the appropriate choice of methodology. Morse & Field (1995, p. 25) identified different types of qualitative questions and linked them with appropriate methodological approaches:

- Chronological or story-oriented questions about the life experiences of an individual and how they unfold over time are often linked with a narrative approach.
- In-depth or descriptive questions focus on developing an in-depth understanding about how different cases, for example individuals, groups or institutions, provide insight into an issue or unique situation. Such questions are frequently linked with a qualitative case study approach (see Chapter 5).
- Process questions about experiences over time, or changes that are characterized by stages and phases, are often linked with grounded theory (see Chapter 4).
- Questions about what is the 'essence' that all persons experience about a specific phenomenon are usually linked with a phenomenological approach (see Chapter 4).
- Community action questions about how changes in practice occur within a community or group can often be linked with a participatory action approach (see Chapter 4).

A good research question or problem is characterized by well-defined terms, relevance to professional and practice concerns, and practicality. Researchers may find themselves forming a broad question initially and focusing it after they begin to generate data (Morse, 2004). For example, 'What is it like to raise a child with cerebral palsy?' opens the researcher to ask about and observe many aspects of family life. Later the question may be narrowed down to, 'How does raising a child with cerebral palsy influence the family's leisure participation?' This example of design flexibility allows the researcher to view phenomena in their entirety and then to recognize the important issues and processes in a particular setting. Locating a setting that is novel to the researcher may heighten awareness and facilitate asking questions of processes and events that might otherwise be accepted implicitly in a more familiar environment. Thus, rehabilitation professionals who work in clinics or hospitals may find it easier, for example, to conduct research at a community center or school.

It may not be feasible to pursue some important research questions given the constraints that researchers may face regarding time, funding, location and recruiting participants. For example, a researcher might be interested in how environments (social, physical, cultural and institutional) shape occupations and what role friendship plays in the health and well-being of people with mood disorders. If, however, the only funding available is to study community participation after discharge from a rehabilitation setting for people with spinal cord injuries, that researcher may develop a question that illuminates the barriers and constraints to community participation related to the environmental factors and relationships.

It may be important to recognize the value-laden nature of health care contexts in the early stages of the research planning process as negotiations may be necessary. It is common for differences in values, beliefs and expected outcomes to exist among the various stakeholders. These stakeholders may include the researcher, the research participants and their respective communities or advocacy groups, and individuals, committees or agencies responsible for approving and/or funding research. The researcher's ability to present cogent reasons for choices made as the research design develops can influence its eventual acceptance.

To understand how values and beliefs can affect research plans, assume that a researcher is interested in the question: 'What are the experiences of recent immigrants using physical therapy services?' This researcher's clinical irritation arises from observing a pattern of limited participation in hospital and outpatient physical therapy by various immigrants who are new to the therapist's home country but who speak English. Having some familiarity with post-colonial theories, as well as intercultural communication concepts, the researcher is unwilling to accept the explanation of "non-compliance" provided by his/her peers and found in the literature. The researcher has strong convictions about equality and fairness and observes discrepancies in health outcomes between people of colour who are immigrants and the "white" people who form the majority. The researcher is also aware that some members of immigrant groups have expressed dissatisfaction with rehabilitation services, but the specific issues are unclear.

The researcher begins to plan an exploratory study that will illuminate the issues, increase understanding, and influence the types and ways in which services are offered. When the researcher presents his/her ideas to the hospital administrators, they frame the problem as "non-compliance" and state that it reflects poorly on their services and limits funding from the government. Based on the belief that the problem lies with the service recipients, the administrators suggest that the provision of translated written materials will resolve the issue. They are interested in documenting increased client visits as the outcome and do not believe that exploring the experiences of immigrants will assist them in achieving that aim. A difference in values and beliefs about the issue is apparent.

Literature that reflects constructivist and critical theorist approaches to the nature of reality, that is, realities are specific to a context, co-constructed and shaped by historical and material conditions (Denzin & Lincoln, 2005), would be consistent with the views held by the researcher. To develop a strong rationale for the importance of this project, the researcher could conduct an initial literature review including physical therapy, occupational therapy and nursing publications. His/her review could include both theoretical writing and research studies, and any departmental and hospital mandates, in order to formulate an argument for this exploratory research.

Conducting a literature review

A literature review is a description of what has been published in peer reviewed journals on the topic of research interest by scholars and researchers. The purpose of a literature review is not just to provide a descriptive account. It should be a critical synthesis of the empirical research and conceptual development related to the topic of interest. The selected literature should be critically appraised in terms of its relevance and the validity and trustworthiness of the research. Conducting a literature review helps to refine the topic of interest or research question and identify gaps in knowledge. Through rigorous review, the researcher determines how the problem has been articulated within and across disciplines, which methodologies have produced useful findings, and whether the topic is worthwhile to study (Morse, 2004). One strategy is to read broadly at first to understand current thinking about a topic and then narrow the focus to research articles. Researchers can begin by identifying key words or phrases to use with databases such as CINAHL, PsycINFO and MEDLINE or by seeking out references noted within key publications. The process of retrieving literature efficiently through the library and other systems will change periodically with technological advances. Developing a good relationship with the local librarian will speed the acquisition part of the literature review process.

The Occupational Therapy Evidence-based Practice Research Group at McMaster University offers a systematic approach to reviewing both qualitative and quantitative research articles through a set of guidelines and accompanying forms (Letts *et al.*, 2007). Alternatively, Morse (2004) suggests making notes on the assumptions made, the knowledge presented and the theoretical stances taken as one reads through each article. Hesse-Biber & Leavy (2006) offer a list of guiding questions for researchers to help review the literature and focus their research topic:

- How have other researchers approached your topic?
- What has been the history of research on this topic?
- What are the research controversies within this literature?
- What specific questions have been asked?
- What has been found out?
- What findings seem most relevant?
- What remains to be done, that is, what burning questions still need to be addressed concerning your topic?
- Where do you find gaps in the literature? (p. 56)

In qualitative research, literature reviews are completed at various junctures in the project in order to serve different purposes. Initially, a literature review helps to clarify the research question and to create an argument for the approval and/or funding of the research. A return to the literature is prompted later by emerging data and the need to construct analytic frameworks that demonstrate how the findings advance theory development (Bogdan & Biklen, 2003). Lastly, a literature review is completed in preparation for dissemination of the research findings. There are different opinions about and practices in the timing and extent of literature reviews; a key concern involves developing preconceived notions that would unduly influence what the researcher is able to discover (Bluff, 2005). Researchers using grounded theory methodology or phenomenology may choose to make explicit their assumptions and then deliberately 'bracket' or set these aside to lessen the chance that the data will match preconceived ideas. Researchers trained in ethnographic methodology are more likely to enter a research setting and begin to generate data prior to any extensive review of the literature (Bogdan & Biklen, 2003). For researchers who are new to the use of literature reviews in qualitative research, the question 'How much literature should I review?' is related to the scope of the project and guidance is usually available from a research supervisor or a more experienced researcher.

Learning more about a topic takes a number of different forms that include talking to researchers and practitioners who have experience with the phenomena of interest. Web sites designed by and for individuals with particular health care conditions such as multiple sclerosis or depression can offer an insider's view of the important issues involved in living with an illness or disability. Less scholarly sources, such as newspaper stories, fiction and memoirs, such as John Hockenberry's *Moving Violations* (1995) or William Styron's *Darkness Visible, a Memoir of Madness* (1990), may also illuminate a topic, sometimes prompting a new perspective of a problem.

Choosing an appropriate research methodology

The term methodology is not used consistently across academic disciplines (Hammell & Carpenter, 2000). In this book we have adopted Hammell's (2006) definition of methodology as 'a specific philosophical and ethical approach to developing knowledge; a theory of how research should, or ought, to proceed given the nature of the issue it seeks to address' (p. 167). The most prevalent methodologies in health care research are *grounded theory*, *phenomenology*, *ethnography* and *participatory action research*, and each of these is discussed in detail in Chapter 4. As we have suggested earlier in this chapter, the type of research question being asked will guide the methodological decision. We do acknowledge, however, that there are no precise definitions of the numerous methodological approaches and the boundaries between them are often blurred (Holloway, 2005). In some situations, where the methodological decision is unclear, researchers may choose to take a more pragmatic approach, and explain and justify their plan of inquiry through reference to the overarching theoretical perspectives associated with qualitative research, such as constructivism, interpretivism and critical theory. As Holloway (2005) said, 'we do not wish to advocate exclusivity or an elitist approach, nor do we see pragmatism as a methodological crime' (p. 101). However, we consider it important that researchers are specific about the approach they adopt in order to avoid the 'unreflexive and undisciplined eclecticism' (Holloway, 2005, p. 101) or methodological blurring that can undermine the rigor and value of qualitative research. An informed and explicitly described methodological approach lends coherence and consistency to the research design, and plays an important role in justifying the plan of inquiry.

Choosing the data collection methods

In order to establish a clear differentiation between 'methods' and 'methodology', we define 'methods as the actual techniques and strategies employed to collect and manipulate data and acquire knowledge' (Hammell & Carpenter, 2000, p. 2).

Interviewing, focus groups, participant observation, consensus techniques and un-obtrusive approaches, such as document analysis of public records and private writings, are the most commonly used methods in health care research, and these are discussed in detail in Chapter 5. These data collection methods have developed from different methodological traditions. For example, participant observation is the anthropologist's main tool in the creation of ethnographic accounts, whereas in-depth interviewing is the phenomenologist's means of generating data to understand lived experience. Baker (cited by Holloway & Todres, 2005, p. 100) describes 'method slurring', that is, the tendency of researchers to cherry pick across methodological traditions without a clear rationale or coherent plan of inquiry. The main question to ask when preparing a research proposal, as suggested by Holloway & Todres (2005), is 'Do the data collection, sampling and analysis pro-cedures "fit" the [research] chosen approach' (p. 101)?

Recruiting participants

Participants are typically involved, selected or recruited through the use of a num-ber of sampling strategies. Broadly defined, sampling strategies are principles and procedures used to identify, choose and gain access to relevant data sources from which data will be generated using the chosen methods (Mason, 2002). The term sampling is often associated solely with the logic derived from the general laws of statistics and probability (Mason, 2002). Probability sampling aims to select a relatively large sample size in a random manner in order to achieve represent-ativeness or determine the degree to which the results can be generalized to a larger population. The logic of probability is not employed in qualitative research. An alternative logic of sampling needs to be established to justify and reinforce the importance of rigorous and systematic approaches to sampling in qualitative research (Mason, 2002; Teddlie & Yu, 2007). As we have discussed earlier in this chapter, qualitative research is primarily exploratory or descriptive rather than explanatory. It focuses on developing in-depth, nuanced understandings of com-plex issues, processes or phenomena. The decision about which sampling strat-egies to use is informed by the research purpose and the methodological approach adopted. These strategies are discussed in detail in Chapter 5. There are, of course, also practical and resource-based issues to consider in making sampling decisions and these will be discussed later in this chapter. In this way, sampling decisions are a combination of theoretical and empirical considerations.

Data management

Qualitative research generates considerable data that are collected using one format and then transferred into another format, usually text-based, for the purposes of storage, retrieval and analysis. The importance of being organized and systematic by creating data management strategies cannot be overstated. Secure data storage is necessary to conform to ethical guidelines. We suggest making copies of all data using multiple technological strategies, for example password protected files on data keys and/or hard drives, and storing these where they cannot be lost, burned or stolen (Patton, 2002). Data are generated using various methods: interviews are audiotaped, participant observations are recorded through field notes, and documents and other materials are collected (Bogdan & Biklen, 2003). The choice of data collection methods directs the researcher to the equipment and human resources that are needed. For example, interviews require a high-quality tape recorder (with a built-in or external microphone), cassette or digital tapes, a transcription machine and a transcriptionist. Basic strategies such as maintaining file folders for printouts of textual data are used despite an increasing reliance on computer-assisted data management and analysis software (Bogdan & Biklen, 2003). Each researcher needs to determine the most comfortable ways of working with the data, either paper copies or on-screen, and incorporate any strategy that will facilitate easy access and manipulation of data. For projects that are small in scope, the choice may be to input data into a word-processing program, print data sets and work with them in a physical way. Increasingly, researchers have been using qualitative software packages that are designed to assist the researcher with retrieving text, coding and retrieving data, and/or developing theory (Patton, 2002). Although it is tempting to think that software programs can analyze data, we emphasize that these programs assist, but it is the researcher who engages in the demanding task of data analysis. Computer assisted qualitative data analysis software (CAQDAS) is a generic term for programs such as NUD*IST, ATLAS.ti and HyperRESEARCH. The practicalities of data management are further explained in Chapter 6.

Data analysis

Data analysis is a systematic process of organizing and presenting data in ways that allow the researcher to make connections, identify patterns and define categories (Bogdan & Biklen, 2003). Qualitative data analysis is based on an interpretive thematic analysis approach that has been further developed within each methodological tradition, for example phenomenology (Colaizzi, 1978), or grounded theory (Strauss & Corbin, 1998). This basic approach to data analysis is described in Chapter 7. It involves a process of data reduction, data display and conclusion drawing and verification (Miles & Huberman, 1994). The data are reduced to manageable units through forms of coding or labelling chunks of text and then displaying these data in new ways. Bogdan & Biklen (2003) describe coding as reviewing the data for evidence of patterns and regularities, topics, events and behaviors and creating categories into which the data fit. This basic data analysis process sounds deceptively simple but in reality it is a time-consuming and intense activity. It involves immersion in the data in order to gain a thorough initial understanding of the data, tracking and recording the decisions made about coding, categories and themes, and consistent reflection about the process and the interpretive decisions being made.

The data will need to be displayed at various stages of the process. Devices used to organize data are primarily visual and physical: concept maps, matrices, diagrams and pictures; coloured post-it notes and papers; highlighter pens, whiteboards and large swaths of newsprint; and index cards. Only one's imagination limits the tools that can be used to engage in displaying the data. It is highly desirable to have a private workspace where work in progress can remain undisturbed. With data managed through word processing or qualitative software programs, multiple copies of text may be reproduced for a variety of visual displays.

Qualitative researchers begin analysis while gathering data, with analysis and interpretation gradually becoming the primary research activities when the data collection ceases (Bogdan & Biklen, 2003). Engaging in some analysis during early stages of the study allows researchers to make changes in the data collection based on what they are learning from participants. It prompts the development of analytic questions and focuses the research. Analyzed data may direct the researcher to observe or ask about a different social process, event or activity. This exemplifies the emergent flexibility inherent in qualitative research design. It is essential for those developing a qualitative research proposal or writing for publication to provide a full account of the data collection and analysis processes.

Strategies for ensuring the study is rigorous

In designing a research project, there are choices that will need to be made to ensure the rigor and trustworthiness of the findings. As Gabard & Martin (2003) suggest, researchers have 'a responsibility to acquire the skills and knowledge to select and implement studies with effective research designs' (p. 233). Trustworthiness, authenticity and credibility are terms that refer to the rigor and quality of qualitative research, that is, the 'truth-value' (Holloway, 2005). Strategies to consider building into the research design include: triangulation, member checking, peer review and an audit trail. As we discussed earlier in this chapter, a number of critical appraisal frameworks (for example Letts *et al.*, 2007) have been developed for evaluating the quality of qualitative research studies and incorporate examples of these strategies. Criteria by which to judge the quality of qualitative research and strategies that can be incorporated into the study design to ensure the rigor of the research will be discussed in Chapter 9.

The role of the researcher

One of the characteristics of qualitative research is the integrated role played by the researcher (Bogdan & Biklen, 2003). Recognition of the researcher's location or social identity (Alcoff, 1991) is part of a process in qualitative research called *reflexivity*, which is discussed in more detail in Chapter 7. An understanding of the researcher's *location* requires a critical examination of how facets of identity such as gender, "race", socio-economic position, education and profession contribute to the research endeavor, including the epistemological claims that are made based on research findings. The research questions we think are valuable, the methodology we choose and the data analysis approach we take are all influenced by the location of the researcher, which is, however, often taken for granted. It is essential that, as researchers, we consistently engage in a critical reflective process, and document this process in the form of field notes and reflective journals during the research process, in order to examine the ways we are privileged and assume positions of power in relation to the research participants. This sort of critical reflection helps researchers determine the extent to which they can 'speak for' rather than 'speak about' people who are vulnerable or who have experienced some form of oppression (Alcoff, 1991). Given the interpretive nature of qualitative research, researchers who develop skills at analyzing and writing about the influence of location on their research are likely to produce trustworthy findings.

Ethical considerations

The value and trustworthiness of research is dependent 'on whether researchers proceed with scientific integrity' (Gabard & Martin, 2003, p. 233). Research ethics is basically concerned with the fundamental issues of informed consent, privacy and confidentiality of data and deception that researchers must identify and address in the initial phase of research design and throughout the project. The Nuremberg Code of 1947 marked the development of modern biomedical research ethics, and later experiments in social sciences and medical research revealed that additional protections were necessary to safeguard the public (Punch, 1994). The infamous research by American psychologist Milgram in the 1960s is a well-known example of how unethical research led to the establishment of principles and practices that are now used in social science and health research (Blass, 2002). Subjects in Milgram's study on authority were deceived into thinking they were providing increasingly painful electric shocks to other subjects, but reassured that the researcher would take responsibility for their decisions. The Tuskegee Syphilis Study (Gray, 1998), a longitudinal study conducted by the US Department of Public Health between 1932 and 1969, involved 400 African-American men infected with syphilis. The purpose was to confirm existing research results on the long-term effects of untreated syphilis. Long after an effective treatment for syphilis was available (in the 1940s), the men were given only aspirin or other placebo treatments to prevent them from obtaining effective treatment. This study not only revealed the racist practices of researchers towards African-Americans, but, like other studies represented an alarming history of abuse and exploitation which overshadowed the indisputable contribution made by research to medical and health care knowledge (Gabard & Martin, 2003). The response to this history has been the development of numerous international and national guidelines (for example the World Medical Association *Declaration of Helsinki*, 2000; the Council for International Organizations of Medical Sciences' *International Ethical Guidelines for Biomedical Research Involving Human Subjects*, 2002) and increasingly formalized processes at national and institutional levels (for example the development of the National Research Ethics Service, formerly the Central Office for Research Ethics Committee in the UK in 2007 and the Medical Research Council of Canada's *Tri-Council Policy Statement for the Ethical Conduct for Research Involving Humans* in 1998).

These guidelines have been influential in developing the independent ethical review processes established by institutions, such as universities or hospitals, which engage in research involving human beings as participants or subjects. Such processes represent an effort to impose ethical standards on research and ensure scientific integrity. These standards are based on a number of ethical principles that we think are worth briefly reviewing before discussing the ethical considerations that need to be addressed when developing a qualitative research proposal and applying for ethics approval.

Scientific integrity is a complex virtue that combines four principles: respect for autonomy, non-maleficence, beneficence and justice (Beauchamp & Childress, 2001). Because the goals of research are to maximize good consequences by discovering new knowledge, rather than to promote the welfare of individual participants, there is a constant danger that researchers will view people as mere means to achieving the aims of the study. The principle of respect for autonomy is central to the concepts of voluntary informed consent and confidentiality. It means that 'the benefits to others must never be won by sacrificing the autonomy of individuals who participate in research' (Gabard & Martin, 2003, p. 227). The principles of non-maleficence (do no harm) and beneficence (promote well-being) relate to protecting potentially vulnerable individuals and groups, minimizing the risks inherent in involvement in the research and enhancing the benefits to the greatest extent possible. Achieving justice is associated with a number of duties inherent in the researcher's role. These duties include ensuring a fair participant recruitment process. As Gabard & Martin (2003) point out, in the past women and minorities have 'been consistently denied inclusion in many research designs' (p. 232). Researchers must identify research priorities and select research topics that are most likely to produce beneficial results in the broader picture as well as for those involved. This duty is encapsulated in Callahan's (cited by Gabard & Martin, 2003) articulation of the Imagination Principle which states that 'researchers have the responsibility to imagine the evil as well as the good ways in which findings might be used' (p. 232). The principle of justice also requires researchers to diligently acquire the skills and knowledge to select and implement studies with appropriate and rigorous research designs in order to ensure the validity and trustworthiness of the findings.

Informed consent requires that potential participants have sufficient information about the nature and objectives of a study to decide whether to participate or not. Despite guidance offered by the principles of respect for autonomy and veracity, there is an art to providing enough information so that individuals are encouraged to volunteer, but not so much detail that it overwhelms or intimidates potential participants. The official format and formal language of informed consent documents may deter individuals who might otherwise participate in the research. Thus, one's attempt to safeguard the public and be transparent about research objectives may cause barriers to recruitment. Information that appears on informed consent forms typically includes an explanation of the participant's role and assurance that it is voluntary; the research methods; the time commitment required; the option to withdraw from participation at any time; the assurance of anonymity; and a description of how the data will be used. The concept of informed consent implicitly assumes that individuals perceive themselves as, and act as, autonomous individuals, which may be contradictory to some worldviews and therefore affect an individual's response to being asked to sign a consent form. Returning to the physical therapy researcher's proposed research with immigrants, what are the possible responses to informed consent forms from these clients? Their responses may be influenced by environmental and personal factors such as educational background, sex, age, previous exposure to research, experience with authority figures, health care perspectives and sense of agency. Illiteracy in the language of the researcher (English, in this case) does not necessarily preclude agreement to participate in research if research assistants can translate the consent form and gather data, for example through interviewing and/or participant observation. Individuals who are marginalized in society or lack political power may feel intimidated by receiving a written consent form from a researcher, who holds a position of authority. Ironically, one measure of informed consent may be when a participant feels able to withdraw from the research and does so.

The emergent nature of qualitative research can also pose a problem in terms of informed consent, as it is not always possible to predict the direction data collection will take, the information obtained or the possible benefits and harms to the participant. Qualitative research is ideally positioned to explore sensitive issues, such as the experience of disability or physical abuse. During interviews, for example, researchers may learn of problems requiring medical intervention; the participant may describe ongoing suicidal thoughts, or have an unexpected psychological response to the questions. The researcher will need to identify a plan that includes referral to an agency or provider that could be available for participants should the need arise and this information should be included in the informed consent documentation (Connelly & Yoder, 2000).

The principle of respect for autonomy requires that a participant's involvement in research is truly voluntary. This means no coercion of any kind, including subtle pressures that come in the form of undue influence (Gabard & Martin, 2003). Undue influence can occur when the researcher is also in a therapeutic relationship with the participant, is in a position of power, for example as an academic conducting research in which students are the participant group, or when participants are offered 'substantial or irresistible tokens of appreciation' (Gabard & Martin, 2003, p. 227). To avoid the appearance of undue influence it is important to devise strategies by which potential participants are initially contacted by someone not involved with the research, provided with information about the study and invited to contact the researcher if interested. All these issues will need to be thoroughly addressed in the research proposal and in completing the ethics review application.

In qualitative research, strategies to ensure research participants' privacy and anonymity range from securely storing all forms of data, for example transcripts, field notes or videotapes, in password protected computer files and locked filing cabinets, to disguising their identities by using pseudonyms in transcripts, field-notes and reports. The transcripts or other data sources should only be made available to members of the research team. The ethic review process also requires that the researcher states how long the data will be kept before being destroyed. The use of a signed contract with the person who transcribes audiotapes is another strategy that helps ensure that data and participants' details remain confidential.

There are a number of reasons, however, why these strategies might be inadequate to ensure anonymity and privacy. The nature of purposive sampling in qualitative research may compromise anonymity if, for example, a limited number of individuals within the researcher's locality meet the research criteria and are known to each other. Research participants may play a significant role in unique, and therefore easily identifiable, organizations such as diagnosis specific advocacy groups. Returning to the example of studying immigrants' experiences with physical therapy, if participants are from a close-knit ethnocultural group, their privacy may be compromised in the analysis process or the final report when the findings are disseminated. To avoid this possibility, researchers may change some key demographic data that do not affect the findings, such as ages of children or job titles.

Confidentiality and anonymity are difficult to maintain when the data collection methods involve the presence of more than one participant, for example when conducting focus groups or engaging in participant observation. 'If informants in a study are members of a small tight-knit group and adequately communicating the findings depends on thick context-embedded descriptions, this will need to be explained to the informants before their agreement to participate' (Connelly & Yoder, 2000, p. 72). When conducting focus groups, Carpenter & Forman (2004), recognizing these difficulties, addressed their concerns about confidentiality with each group, set ground rules about the group's interaction and asked the participants to use only first names. They also offered to send the focus group transcripts to each participant so they had the opportunity to delete (or add) any information they wished before the data were analyzed.

Deception occurs when the investigator fails to reveal the research intent and objectives (Hesse-Biber & Leavy, 2006). Misrepresentation of oneself and the omission of vested interests also constitute deception. Issues such as the researcher pretending to be a member of the group, feigning beliefs or engaging in activities to fit into a research setting, for example smoking when one is a non-smoker, have the potential to affect the research relationship negatively if participants become aware of these small deceptions.

The ethical principles of respect for autonomy, beneficence, non-maleficence and justice represent universal values and are embodied in the ethics review standards established by clinical, professional and academic institutions. However, these standards were developed as a means of scrutinizing and monitoring quantitative research projects and, as a result, protection of the research "subject", informed consent, confidentiality and anonymity have been identified as primary ethical issues.

Ethical considerations encountered in qualitative research are more wide-ranging and ongoing in nature. 'They are empirical and theoretical and *permeate* the qualitative research process' (Mauthner *et al.*, 2002, p. 1), and reflect the flexible nature of qualitative research and the central role of the researcher as *research instrument* that we will discuss in subsequent chapters. The notion that the 'tricky' ethical issues associated with qualitative research 'can be handled by a single set of universal standards (embodied in a legal sounding document) is itself problematic' (Mattingly, 2005, p. 455). These problems have been exacerbated by a lack of understanding among research ethics committee members of qualitative methodological approaches and their implications (Mauthner *et al.*, 2002; Khanou & Peter, 2005; Mattingly, 2005; Walker *et al.*, 2005). It is our experience that research ethics committees are beginning to review qualitative research submissions in ways that reflect an increasing understanding of the unique characteristics of specific methodologies. Qualitative research authors (for example Sandelowski *et al.* 1989; Connelly & Yoder, 2000; Kuzel *et al.*, 2003; Walker *et al.*, 2005) have also recognized the need to provide guidance in developing successful qualitative research proposals for ethics review or funding agencies.

Practical issues

Timelines

The maxim that research always takes longer than a researcher thinks is confirmed by Morse's (2004) expert advice: 'estimate the amount of time you think the project will take, and then double it!' (p. 498). Morse suggests that approximately three months is needed to conceptualize and write a qualitative research proposal. The proposal includes all the components introduced in this chapter. The ethics approval process, whether academic or health care institution or both, often involves the researcher addressing provisos or changes that the committee requires before approval is granted. Public and private funding bodies have proposal submission deadlines and may require ethical approval for the research from the primary investigator's place of employment, for example a hospital or university.

For research with potentially vulnerable and marginalized groups of people, and in some contexts immigrants receiving rehabilitation services fit this description, it is necessary to budget additional time to complete the research. Meadows *et al.* (2003) conduct research with immigrant, First Nations and women's groups and they value taking time to work with participants to address ethical and cultural issues as they arise. One of their recommendations is that 'timelines must reflect the need for community consultation, recruitment and/or training of researcher(s) within the community, and multi-stage processes of consent' (p. 18). This advice is particularly applicable to planning and implementing participatory action research, as negotiation, building relationships and consensus are integral features of this approach.

Budget

A well-designed research proposal helps to identify what services, supplies and equipment are needed to complete the research within the timeline established. The scope of the project, including sample size, data generation methods and analytic strategies, and the extent to which the researcher has release time from other responsibilities, all influence the types of expenses that are reasonable to present for funding. Typical categories of expenses in a university and community-partnered rehabilitation study are: personnel; equipment and supplies; services; overhead and infrastructure; and travel. Personnel include a research assistant, a research coordinator and the primary investigator, who may be eligible to receive some salary support. Examples of research equipment are digital or audio recorders, transcription machines, computers, printers and filing cabinets. Supplies are expendable and include copying and printing costs, paper, mailing (postage, envelopes, letterhead stationery), files and long-distance telephone charges. Services for a mixed methods research design may include consultation with a statistician, and if interviews are used to gather data, a person is needed to transcribe the audiotapes. Overhead and infrastructure refer to staff services and research space that the health care agency, university and/or community organization provide. Travel to conferences for the purpose of presenting the research findings is a reasonable expense to budget. Creating a realistic budget is a relatively straightforward task and is a key component of proposals that are submitted to funding bodies.

Preparing and organizing

The practicalities of doing qualitative research are influenced by the researcher's work or academic environment, the level of support available there, their organizational skills and good luck. Academic environments offer mentorship and support in the form of research supervisors and other students at different stages of learning about qualitative research. We recommend joining a qualitative research interest group, either online or face to face, as this provides a venue for working through ideas for proposals and making methodological decisions. Online groups offer the opportunity to learn about qualitative research by reading the postings or posing questions to which others can respond. Current online discussion groups may be located by using popular Internet search engines. A research mentor will help you to develop your ideas, review the proposal and ethics application and share research experiences. It is often through hearing others' mistakes that we learn what works well.

The process of *entering the field* refers to finding a research setting and recruiting participants for the study. In order to find a suitable research setting, the researchers may need to use any contacts they have. Finding the *gatekeeper* to desired setting is one of the first steps; this person can provide information about how best to present the study to the people responsible for approving the research in a particular setting. For example, after Suto (2000) made several 'cold calls' to board and care homes to describe her proposed study, a member of her supervisory committee referred her to an acquaintance of his who owned this kind of sheltered housing. She wrote a letter to the facility owner outlining plans for her research, requested an interview and subsequently presented her research plans to residents of the facility for their approval after receiving the owner's support. Writing flyers to advertise the study, preparing presentations and written materials for different levels of understanding and/or literacy, and talking with participants are all activities of entering the field. It is challenging to synthesize a lengthy and formally written document (the research proposal) and create a short presentation for potential participants and colleagues who may offer recruitment leads. Good organizational skills are beneficial as they assist in balancing the demands of work and research responsibilities, scheduling interviews, managing data and in some cases providing training to research staff. If interviews are the data gathering method, it is important to consider where they will occur. The advantages and disadvantages of interviewing participants in institutional settings such as hospitals, universities and rehabilitation clinics need to be considered; sometimes these settings make it harder for the participants to view a clinician who has provided rehabilitation services as a researcher. Attention to small details enhances the data gathering and increases self-confidence.

If hiring a transcriptionist, it is important to anticipate the time required to hire and supervise that person. Larger and well-funded research projects may allow for the hiring and/or supervising of research assistants to collect data and a project coordinator to manage the study. Time must be allocated for purchasing equipment and supplies, setting up the research area, learning to use the equipment, for example voice recognition software, contacting participants and engaging in other unforeseen research tasks.

Dissemination of research findings

Qualitative research findings are a type of evidence that may be used to guide physical therapy and occupational therapy theories, inform curricula and be incorporated into practice (Hammell, 2004). The final research report or account builds on writing that the researcher has done periodically during the research process, for example when presenting research in progress at a seminar or team meeting (Holloway, 2005). A plan of how the research findings will potentially be disseminated needs to be developed for inclusion in the proposal and ethics approval application. In formulating this plan there are a number of questions to consider. First, who are the different audiences who will read the account? Ideally, occupational therapy and physical therapy researchers will publish in peer-reviewed journals for practitioners and academics in their respective professions. The topics addressed by qualitative research approaches are frequently of interest to an interdisciplinary audience and, as such, may also be published in different journals that other health care professionals read. Second, what is most important to present in these different types of reports? Some research accounts have a strong theoretical focus and the participants' voices may be less prominent than the researcher's interpretive voice. For research where empowerment is one of the main goals, the researcher may craft the report to highlight the participants' perspectives. Third, where and how should the findings be disseminated? Beyond peer-reviewed journals, researchers can present their findings via teleconferences, in verbal and poster presentations at conferences and in 'rounds' within hospital settings. It is challenging to present qualitative research accounts effectively at professional conferences that allot 10 or 15 minutes per paper and in these instances, focusing on a particular aspect of the report may be most appropriate. The dissemination of qualitative research findings raises some controversial and ethical issues and these will be discussed in Chapter 8.

In this chapter we have outlined the essential components – theoretical, ethical and practical – that need to be considered when planning a qualitative research study, developing a proposal, completing an ethics approval submission, and applying for funding. A number of these components will be discussed in more depth in Chapters 5–8. In the next chapter, we will discuss four methodological approaches to qualitative research that are commonly employed in health research, and the importance of matching these with the substantive issue being investigated.

References

Alcoff, L. (1991) The problem of speaking for others. *Cultural Critique, 20* (Winter), 5–32.

Beauchamp, T.L. & Childress, J.F. (2001) *Principles of Biomedical Ethics* (5th edn). New York, Oxford University Press.

Blass, T. (2002) The man who shocked the world. *Psychology Today, 35* (2), 68–75.

Bluff, R. (2005) Grounded theory: the methodology. In: I. Holloway (ed.), *Qualitative Research in Health Care* (pp. 147–167). Maidenhead, UK, Open University Press.

Bogdan, R.C. & Biklen, S.K. (2003) *Qualitative Research for Education: an Introduction to Theory and Methods* (4th edn). Boston, Allyn & Bacon.

Brown, G.A. (2006) Grounded theory and sensitizing concepts. *International Journal of Qualitative Methods, 5* (3), Article 2. Retrieved 10 January 2007 from: http://www.ualberta.ca/~ijqm/backissues/5_3/pdf/bowen

Carpenter, C. (2000). Exploring the lived experience of disability. In: K.W. Hammell, C. Carpenter & I. Dyck (eds), *Using Qualitative Research: a Practical Introduction for Occupational and Physical Therapists* (pp. 23–33). Edinburgh, Churchill Livingstone.

Carpenter, C. & Forman, B. (2004) Provision of community programs for clients with spinal cord injury: using qualitative research to evaluate the role of the British Columbia Paraplegic Association. *Topics in Spinal Cord Injury Rehabilitation, 9* (4), 57–72.

Colaizzi, P.F. (1978) Psychological research as the phenomenologist views it. In: R.S. Valle & M. King (eds), *Existential Phenomenological Alternatives for Psychology* (pp. 48–71). New York, Oxford University Press.

Connelly, L. & Yoder, L. (2000) Improving qualitative proposals: common problem areas. *Clinical Nurse Specialist, 14* (2), 69–74.

Corring, D. & Cook, J.V. (1999) Client-centered care means that I am a valued human being. *Canadian Journal of Occupational Therapy, 66* (2), 71–82.

Council for International Organizations of Medical Sciences (CIOMS) (2002) *International Ethical Guidelines for Biomedical Research Involving Human Subjects.*

Geneva, World Health Organization. Retrieved 12 March 2007 from: http://www.cioms.ch/frame_guidelines_nov_2002.htm

Creswell, J., Hanson, W.E., Clark, V.L.P. & Morales, A. (2007) Qualitative research designs: selection and implementation. *The Counselling Psychologist*, 35 (2), 236–264.

Denzin, N.K. & Lincoln, Y.S. (2005) Introduction: the discipline and practice of qualitative research. In: N.K. Denzin & Y.S. Lincoln (eds), *The Sage Handbook of Qualitative Research* (3rd edn, pp. 1–32). Thousand Oaks, Calif., Sage.

Gabard, D. & Martin, M. (2003) *Physical Therapy Ethics*. Philadelphia, F.A. Davis.

Geertz, C. (1973) *The Interpretation of Cultures: Selected Essays*. New York, Basic Books.

Gray, F.D. (1998) *The Tuskegee Syphilis Study: the Real Story and Beyond*. Montgomery, Ala., New South Books.

Hammell, K.W. (2004) Quality of life among people with high spinal cord injury living in the community. *Spinal Cord*, 42 (11), 607–620.

Hammell, K.W. (2006) *Perspectives on Disability and Rehabilitation: Contesting Assumptions, Challenging Practice*. Edinburgh, Churchill Livingstone/Elsevier.

Hammell, K.W. & Carpenter, C. (2000) Introduction to qualitative research in occupational therapy and physical therapy. In: K.W. Hammell, C. Carpenter & I. Dyck (eds), *Using Qualitative Research: a Practical Introduction for Occupational and Physical Therapists* (pp. 1–12). Edinburgh, Churchill Livingstone.

Hammersley, M. & Atkinson, P. (1995) *Ethnography: Principles in Practice* (2nd edn). London, Routledge & Kegan Paul.

Hesse-Biber, S.N. & Leavy, P. (2006) *The Practice of Qualitative Research*. Thousand Oaks, Calif., Sage.

Hockenberry, J. (1995) *Moving Violations*. New York, Hyperion.

Holloway, I. (2005) Qualitative writing. In: I. Holloway (ed.), *Qualitative Research in Health Care* (pp. 270–286). Maidenhead, UK, Open University Press.

Holloway, I. & Todres, L. (2005) The status of method: flexibility, consistency and coherence. In: I. Holloway (ed.), *Qualitative Research in Health Care* (pp. 90–103). Maidenhead, UK, Open University Press.

Khanou, N. & Peter, E. (2005) Participatory action research: considerations for ethical review. *Social Science & Medicine*, 60, 2333–2340.

Kuzel, A.J., Woolf, S.H., Engel, J.D. *et al.* (2003) Making the case for a qualitative study of medical errors in primary care. *Qualitative Health Research*, 13 (6), 743–780.

Letts, L., Wilkins, S., Law, M., Stewart, D., Bosch, J. & Westmorland, M. (2007) *Guidelines for Critical Review Form: Qualitative Studies (Version 2.0)*. Hamilton, McMaster University. Retrieved 12 January 2007 from: http://www.fhs.mcmaster.ca/rehab/ebp/

Mason, J. (2002) *Qualitative Researching* (2nd edn). London, Sage.

Mattingly, C. (2005) Toward a vulnerable ethics of research practice. *Health: an Interdisciplinary Journal of the Social Study of Health, Illness and Medicine*, 9 (4), 453–471.

Mauthner, M., Birch, M., Jessop, J. & Miller, T. (2002) *Ethics in Qualitative Research*. London, Sage.

Meadows, L.M., Lagendyk, L.E., Thurston, W.E. & Eisener, A.C. (2003) Balancing culture, ethics and methods in qualitative health research with Aboriginal peoples. *International Journal of Qualitative Methods*, 2 (4). Retrieved 3 January 2007 from: http://www.ualberta.ca/~iiqm/backissues/2_4/pdf/meadows.pdf

Medical Research Council of Canada (1998) *Tri-Council Policy Statement for the Ethical Conduct of Research Involving Humans in Canada*. Retrieved 12 March 2007 from: http://www.pre.ethics.gc.ca/english/pdf/TCPS%20June2003_E.pdf

Miles, M.B. & Huberman, A.M. (1994) *Qualitative Data Analysis* (2nd edn). Thousand Oaks, Calif., Sage.

Morse, J.M. (2004) Preparing and evaluating qualitative research proposals. In: C. Seale, G. Gobo, J.F. Gubrium & D. Silverman (eds), *Qualitative Research Practice* (pp. 493–503). Thousand Oaks, Calif., Sage.

Morse, J.M. & Field, P.A. (1995) *Qualitative Research Methods for Health Professionals* (2nd edn). Thousand Oaks, Calif., Sage.

Morse, J.M. & Richards, L. (2002). *Read Me First for a User's Guide to Qualitative Methods.* Thousand Oaks, Calif., Sage.

National Research Ethics Service (2007) London. Retrieved 25 June 2007 from: http://www.nres.npsa,nhs.uk/

Patton, M.Q. (2002) *Qualitative Research & Evaluation Methods* (3rd edn). Thousand Oaks, Calif., Sage.

Punch, M. (1994) Politics and ethics in qualitative research. In: N.K. Denzin & Y.S. Lincoln (eds), *Handbook of Qualitative Research* (pp. 83–97). Thousand Oaks, Calif., Sage.

Richardson, B. (2006) An ethnography of physiotherapy culture. In: L. Finlay & C. Ballinger (eds), *Qualitative Research for Allied Health Professionals: Challenging Choices* (pp. 79–92). Chichester, UK, Whurr Publications.

Sandelowski, M., Davis, D. & Harris, B. (1989) Artful design: writing the proposal for research in the naturalist paradigm. *Research in Nursing & Health*, *12*, 77–84.

Sim, J. & Wright, C. (2000) *Research in Health Care: Concepts, Designs and Methods.* Cheltenham, Nelson Thomas.

Strauss, A. & Corbin, J. (1998) *Basics of Qualitative Research: Techniques and Procedures for Developing Grounded Theory.* Thousand Oaks, Calif., Sage.

Styron, W. (1990) *Darkness Visible: a Memoir of Madness.* New York, Random House.

Suto, M. (2000) Issues related to data collection. In: K.W. Hammell, C. Carpenter & I. Dyck (eds), *Using Qualitative Research: a Practical Introduction for Occupational and Physical Therapists* (pp. 35–46). Edinburgh, Churchill Livingstone.

Teddlie, C. & Yu, F. (2007) Mixed method sampling: a typology with examples. *Journal of Mixed Methods Research*, *1* (1), 77–100.

Walker, J., Holloway, I. & Wheeler, S. (2005) Guidelines for ethical review of qualitative research. *Research Ethics Review*, *1* (3), 90–96.

World Medical Association (2000) Declaration of Helsinki: Ethical Principles for Medical Research Involving Human Subjects. Retrieved 10 March 2007 from: http://www.wma.net/e/policy/b3.htm

Chapter 4

USING METHODOLOGICAL THEORY IN PLANNING QUALITATIVE RESEARCH

Introduction

In Chapter 1, we discussed the theoretical context of rehabilitation within which research conducted by occupational therapists and physical therapists can be located and how the influence of theories and models of disability and rehabilitation on practice and research needs to be reflected upon and made explicit. Theory is also integral to the practice of research in health care. Each researcher approaches the research – whether qualitative or quantitative paradigms – from a unique ontological position that specifies the research question or issue to be addressed, that is, the knowledge that is being sought (epistemology) which is then investigated by employing a specific research approach (methodology). As discussed in Chapter 1, 'when qualitative research is conducted without reference to theoretical frameworks, the researcher effectively takes for granted a particular framework without acknowledging it' (Rice & Ezzy, 1999, p. 10). This is problematic if the desired outcome of the research is the discovery of new insights or knowledge about an issue.

A *paradigm* can be defined as a 'basic set of beliefs that guide action and are shared by a scientific community' (Denzin & Lincoln, 2005, p. 22). The quantitative paradigm, informed by a philosophy of positivism, has come to be known as the traditional research approach to scientific inquiry. The ontological and epistemological assumptions that underpin this paradigm are implicit and rarely questioned by those engaged in quantitative research. Qualitative research, in contrast, 'has no theory or paradigm that is distinctly its own' (Denzin & Lincoln, 2005, p. 22); rather, it is informed by a number of philosophical systems, for example interpretivism, constructivism, hermeneutics and critical theory, which we introduced in Chapter 2. This 'multiparadigmatic' (Denzin & Lincoln, 2005, p. 7) nature is reflected in the various methodological theories that are associated with qualitative inquiry. This chapter will introduce some of the methodological theories (diversely, and somewhat confusingly, called methodological orientations, approaches, strategies and philosophical traditions in the literature) that have informed and influenced the design and implementation of qualitative research.

Methodological theories in qualitative research

In this chapter, we will discuss the methodologies most commonly represented in the health care literature, in terms of their characteristic concepts or key ideas, in order to illuminate how they might be used in rehabilitation research. These methodologies are grounded theory, phenomenology, ethnography and participatory action research. Creswell (1998) observed that 'those undertaking qualitative studies have a baffling number' of [methodological] traditions from which to choose (p. 4) and there are notably different interpretations or 'subfields' of methodological theories or traditions, for example hermeneutics or descriptive phenomenology. In this book, we have followed Creswell's (1998) example and focused on the work of certain influential proponents of the different methodological approaches being described.

Grounded theory

Grounded theory has proved to be one of the most influential approaches to qualitative inquiry, particularly in nursing, and key features of grounded theory are often adapted to meet the needs of other approaches. Concerns have been raised (Strauss & Corbin, 1994) that, as a consequence, researchers lack understanding of the original logic and purpose of grounded theory. Glaser & Strauss first developed the grounded theory approach in their pioneering book *The Discovery of Grounded Theory* (1967). It represented a melding of their research backgrounds in their collaborative exploration of the experience of patients dying in hospital (Glaser & Strauss, 1968). Glaser's background as a quantitative researcher was combined with Strauss's training in field research and symbolic interactionism. As a result, grounded theory can be situated closer to the quantitative paradigm than any other qualitative approach. It combines assumptions of an objective and external reality with unbiased data collection conducted by a neutral observer. It uses reductionist procedures to manage data and seeks a theoretical outcome that can be subsequently tested and verified. At the same time, the authors recognized the issues of *giving voice* to the participants, representing them as accurately as possible and the interpretive (creative) nature of the data analysis process. Thus, grounded theory can be considered both deductive and inductive (Charmaz, 2000; Bluff, 2005).

Since the publication of Glaser's book *Basics of Grounded Theory Analysis: Emergence vs Forcing* (1992), in which he vociferously criticized the approach taken by Strauss in collaboration with Corbin (Strauss & Corbin, 1990), the development of grounded theory has been characterized by the public debate between these proponents of grounded theory. The main issue focused on Glaser's criticism that Strauss & Corbin had deviated from the original intent of grounded theory in developing a detailed, systematic and, in his opinion, more prescriptive "scientific" approach to data analysis that 'forces' the development of theory (Charmaz, 2000). This debate may have contributed to confusion about the data analysis procedures and aim of this research approach (Strauss & Corbin, 1994).

There are, however, a number of key features that clearly differentiate grounded theory from other qualitative methodologies.

Grounded theory is primarily a systematic analytic approach to the 'generation or discovery of a [substantive] theory, an abstract analytical schema of a phenomenon that relates to a particular situation' (Creswell, 1998, p. 56). The purpose of such theories is to make explicit the reality of how people perceive particular situations in the context of their environment and culture and the way they interact and communicate with each other (Bluff, 2005). The theory is articulated toward the end of the study and can assume the form of a narrative statement, a graphic presentation, or a series of hypotheses or propositions (Creswell, 1998). The research question or aim basically identifies the phenomenon to be studied and is initially broad, for example Rose *et al.* (2002) were guided by the question: 'How do families respond to mental illness in the social and interpersonal contexts of their daily lives?' The outcome of their research was the development of a grounded theory of pursuing normalcy that illuminated the complex and difficult process of integrating the social implications and personal interpretations of mental illness. Schachter *et al.* (1999) were guided by the aim to explore the reactions of women survivors of childhood abuse to physical therapy and their ideas about physical therapy that would be sensitive to their needs. The authors developed a theory that encompassed survivors' experiences and ideas for sensitive practices, which, after further study phases, resulted in the development of the *Handbook of Sensitive Practice for Health Professionals* (Schachter *et al.*, 2001).

The key features of grounded theory focus on analytic strategies, not sampling and data collection methods (Charmaz, 2000). In grounded theory, the same methods as other qualitative inquiry approaches are used and these will be discussed in more detail in the next chapter. Grounded theory offers 'researchers a set of clear guidelines from which to build explanatory frameworks that specify relationships' (Charmaz, 2000, p. 510). The systematic nature of the data analysis process and the procedural strategies are attractive to some researchers and, in particular, for those with less experience in qualitative inquiry. The data analysis process can begin as data are being collected and certainly soon after the interviews are transcribed or observations conducted (Bluff, 2005). Creswell (1998) visualizes the linkages between data collection and analysis in grounded theory as a zigzag process: 'out to the field to gather information, analyze the data, back to the field to gather more information, analyze the data, and so forth' (p. 57). This simultaneous and interactive process is called the *constant comparative method*, the purpose of which is to identify similarities and differences in the data (words, sentences, paragraphs, codes and categories) at all levels of the analysis process (Bluff, 2005). This means, for example, comparing different people (such as their views, situations, actions, accounts and experiences), comparing data from the same individual at different points of time, comparing incident with incident, comparing data with categories and comparing a category with other categories (Charmaz, 2000, p. 515). This process continues until the final report is written and enables the researcher to gain a thorough understanding of the phenomenon being studied.

The core concept of the analysis process in grounded theory is *coding*. Initial or *open coding* represents the initial phase and proceeds by examining the data line by line. During this phase, actions and events revealed in the data are defined (Charmaz, 2000), questions are generated and answers sought in the participants' own words. These questions, if likely to facilitate the development of theory, can be asked of future participants and these 'can also generate working hypotheses or propositions that can be validated in subsequent data collection' (Bluff, 2005, p. 154). *Line-by-line coding* draws the researcher's attention to *sensitizing concepts*, that is, 'background ideas that inform the overall research problem' (Charmaz, 2000, p. 515). These ideas are derived from the researcher's theoretical and professional perspectives; for example, Charmaz's work in exploring the experiences of chronic illness was informed by sociology and the theoretical concepts of self and identity.

Codes with similar meanings or definitions are linked together to form a *category*, which is a method of abstracting the data from the participants' overall accounts. The approaches of Glaser (1992) and Strauss & Corbin (1998) to coding are similar, but Strauss & Corbin adopted more detailed procedures that they defined as: dimensionalization, axial coding, selective coding and the conditional matrix. The process of *dimensionalization* involves locating a category along a continuum, according to its characteristic or property. Rose *et al.* (2002) identified how participants conceptualized mental illness on a continuum: as biologically based at one end of the continuum and in terms of normal behavior at the other end. *Axial coding*, which generally follows open coding, can be perceived as the next phase or Level 2 coding. Axial coding is aimed at making connections between categories, including conditions that give rise to the category, its context, the social interactions within it and its consequences (Charmaz, 2000). Through this process, the researcher can identify a *core category* that is central to the phenomenon being studied, which links the data and accounts for variations in the data (Strauss & Corbin, 1998). At this stage some of the open codes may be discarded because no connections can be established, but *negative cases* are retained (Bluff, 2005) as these will further direct data collection. Strauss & Corbin (1998) described a further strategy called *selective coding*, intended to link the categories and sub-categories to the core category. In this process, the researcher identifies an emergent storyline and writes a narrative description that integrates the categories established through the axial coding process (Creswell, 1998). These connections or storylines can be visually portrayed as a *conditional matrix*. Strauss & Corbin (1990) describe the conditional matrix as an analytic diagram that maps the social, historical and economic conditions and consequences related to the core category or phenomenon being studied. According to Creswell (1998), 'this phase of analysis is not frequently found in most grounded theory studies' (p. 57).

The ability of the researcher to give meaning to the data, that is, to recognize what is relevant and important for the emerging theory, what is missing and what informs the phenomenon being studied, requires *theoretical sensitivity* (Bluff, 2005). It is this ability that facilitates another key feature of grounded theory – *theoretical sampling* – where data analysis informs the sampling selection, which may be based on the need to access participants with specific information or experiences, or to develop or confirm emerging concepts (Bluff, 2005). The aim of *theoretical sampling* is to refine ideas, not to increase the size of the sample, and is a pivotal component of formal theory development (Charmaz, 2000). Charmaz (2000) recommends *theoretical sampling* later in the research process, 'in order that relevant data and analytic directions emerge without being forced' (p. 520). In grounded theory, data saturation is linked to theoretical sampling and is said to occur 'when each category is conceptually dense, variations in the category have been identified and explained, and no further data pertinent to the categories emerge during data collection' (Bluff, 2005, p. 155). Some authors (Morse, 1995; Charmaz, 2000) consider that, in reality, saturation is a difficult concept to nail down, that it is not possible to fully saturate the data, and that data collection is curtailed more by the practical constraints of conducting research in the 'real world'.

Analytic memos or notes are the written records researchers keep to record their abstract thinking about data (Hammersley & Atkinson, 1995) and these are considered an important tool in grounded theory. According to Charmaz (2000) memo writing:

> Helps researchers (a) to grapple with ideas about the data, (b) to set an analytic course, (c) to refine categories [of information about the phenomenon within the data], (d) to define relationships among various categories, and (e) to gain a sense of confidence and competence in their ability to analyze data (pp. 517–518).

In summary, grounded theory refers both to the approach to inquiry and to the product of inquiry, but researchers commonly use the term to mean a systematic mode of analysis (Charmaz, 2005). A grounded theory is developed through a complex and time-consuming zigzag process that, if the emerging theory is to have applicability and credibility, requires considerable dedication and commitment on the part of the researcher. Inherent in the grounded theory approach is 'a set of flexible, yet rigorous, analytic guidelines that enable researchers to focus their data collection and to build inductive middle-range theories through successive levels of data analysis and conceptual development' (Charmaz, 2005, p. 507). The development of grounded theory has had a significant influence on qualitative inquiry and many of the concepts associated with this methodology have been co-opted by other approaches. This makes it all the more important that researchers, when undertaking a grounded theory study, make explicit the approach they have adopted (Bluff, 2005).

Phenomenology

The word 'phenomenon' has its origins in the Greek term *phaenesthai*, meaning 'to show itself' or 'to appear'. Edmond Husserl (1859–1938) developed phenomenology in the early 1900s as a rigorous philosophical approach to revealing the intelligibility of human experience as a source of study in its own right. The advent of phenomenology raised some important epistemological issues and questioned the foundation and status of knowledge, including questions such as: 'What is "real" and "valid?" ' 'What constitutes "evidence?" ' and 'What is the relationship between the "knower" and the "known?" ' A number of philosophers and theorists, for example Heidegger, Gadamer, Schutz and Merleau-Ponty, have further developed phenomenology and moved it in different directions, for example Merleau-Ponty's (1962) existential phenomenology and Schutz's (1972) social or interpretive phenomenology. These theorists offered little in the way of empirical or practical guidance for conducting phenomenological research. In recent years, a number of authors have attempted to address this problem, for example Giorgi (1985), Moustakas (1994) and van Manen (1990). Empirical phenomenology 'involves a return to experience in order to obtain comprehensive descriptions that provide the basis for a reflective structural analysis that portrays the essences of the experience' (Moustakas, 1994, p. 13).

The complexity of the ideas and philosophical concepts embedded in phenomenology are, however, challenging and difficult to comprehend fully, particularly for those of us with no philosophical background. Despite these difficulties, there is a growing interest in this methodological approach to understanding, describing and interpreting human behavior and experience in health care research. Two approaches in particular are influential in health care: descriptive phenomenology and hermeneutic or interpretive phenomenology. Descriptive phenomenologists, for example Giorgi (1997, 2003a, 2003b) and Moustakas (1994), have perhaps the closest connections with Husserl's original conception of phenomenology and focus on creating detailed descriptions of the specific experiences of others. *Descriptive phenomenology* involves a disciplined procedure designed to ensure that the intrinsic meaning of the narratives is faithfully presented (Todres, 2005). The overall goal is a goodness of fit between the researcher's 'general formulations and the specific details of the text and how they interrelate' (Todres, 2005, p. 111). *Interpretive or hermeneutic phenomenologists*, for example van Manen (1990, 1997), emphasize the ordinary language of everyday experience and seek 'to understand the nature of human beings and the meanings they bestow upon the world by examining language in its cultural context; the way language is given meaning and interpreted' (Rapport, 2005, p. 125). The belief that humans are self-determining beings is a core characteristic of interpretive phenomenology and, as such, participants contribute their own interpretations of their experiences to the 'hermeneutic conversation' (Rapport, 2005, p. 135). The term *hermeneutic* describes the process of establishing understanding of a text as a whole by constantly interpreting the individual parts in relation to the other parts and each in relation to the whole. The circular nature of this form of interpretive analysis emphasizes the importance of the cultural, historical and social context in identifying meaning. Hermeneutics is a central feature of phenomenological data analysis.

It is not possible, within this chapter, to do justice to the core philosophical ideas of these evolving approaches. We have provided important references for those readers who would like to explore these approaches in more depth and engage in the academic debates about the splits between the different types of phenomenology. There are, however, a number of core concepts and principles characteristic of the phenomenological approach to research.

Central to the phenomenological research endeavor is the search for the central underlying meaning of the experience or phenomenon described as the *essence*, 'the essential, invariant structure' (Creswell, 1998, p. 52). 'The goal of phenomenology is to uncover commonalities and differences not private idiosyncratic events of understandings' (Benner, 1994, p. 104). Researchers are interested in understanding what human conditions and commonalities make the distinctions and differences possible. The concept of *essence* can be explained by considering the phenomena of 'love' or the experience of the colour 'blue'. In spite of the unique variations and contexts of these phenomena, people who experience them consistently recognize them and share that recognition with others. Experiences of phenomena have an underlying structure, for example the phenomena of 'grief' can be described, whether the loved one is a dog, a parrot or a child (Creswell, 1998). The *essence* of a phenomenon thus refers to 'the qualities that give an experiential phenomenon its distinctiveness and coherence' (Todres 2005, p. 105). The *essential structure* of a phenomenon emphasizes the *intentionality of consciousness* 'where experiences contain both external appearance and inward consciousness based on memory, image, and the meaning [attributed to it]' (Creswell, 1998, p. 52). This concept of *intentionality* relates to the assumption that the *life world* 'is not an objective environment or a subjective consciousness or set of beliefs; rather, [it] is what we perceive and experience it to be' (Finlay, 1999, p. 302). It highlights the idea of *multiple realities*, that the same objects or situations can mean different things to different people, and that people and the worlds they occupy are inextricably intertwined. In this way, phenomenologists focus on the *life world*, which, according to Husserl, is the source of all experiential qualities. The terms 'love' and 'blue' would have no meaning without the 'reality' in which we live. This 'reality' is both 'the world of objects around us as we perceive them, and our experiences of our self, body and relationships' (Finlay, 1999, p. 301).

The research process is based on two additional principles that are characteristic of phenomenology: *phenomenological reduction* and *bracketing*. Phenomenology is fundamentally committed to describing, not explaining, how and why meanings arise, 'to give plausible insight rather than attempt to develop a theory' (Finlay, 1999, p. 301). This is achieved through a process of *phenomenological reduction*, whereby the data are searched for all possible meanings and descriptions of emerging categories and themes are formulated. In phenomenological research, the aim is to gain rich and 'thick' information which 'communicates the sense and logic of the phenomenon to others' (Todres, 2005, p. 110). This usually entails recruiting a small number of participants using a purposive sampling strategy. Data are collected through one or two extensive semi-structured interviews with each participant. A full description is articulated of the participants' contexts and experiences (Todres, 2005). A number of approaches to data analysis have been developed within phenomenology (Giorgi, 1985, 1997; Smith, 2003) and these will be discussed in more detail in Chapter 7.

Phenomenological reduction is predicated on the concept of *bracketing* or *epoche*, meaning to suspend all judgments – presuppositions, interpretations, and prior knowledge and understanding – in order to enter the unique world of the individual whose experience is being studied. The aim is to listen genuinely and actively to the participant's perspective, 'to experience the process of discovering the phenomenon first hand through direct contact or intuition' (Finlay, 1999, p. 302) and to see the world from the other person's point of view. It is, of course, impossible to *bracket* fully the prior knowledge and assumptions one brings to the research process. Our prior knowledge contributes to the development of relevant research questions, choice of a methodology and study design decisions. The key is for researchers to reflect critically on the beliefs, values and assumptions they have about the phenomenon and why they think the questions they are asking are relevant (Benner, 1994).

In summary, the aim of phenomenology is to reveal the individual's lived meaning of the world; it does not assume an understanding, but rather works at developing it, using the terms of meaning constructed by the participant. The emphasis is on researchers bracketing their own presuppositions and understandings of the phenomenon in order to enter the participants' life world fully. Through a rigorous, interpretive data analysis process the essential features of a phenomenon are revealed, which can then be fully and non-judgmentally described for others. An example is provided by Carpenter's (1994) study, which sought to understand the experience of traumatic spinal cord injury from the perspective of individuals who defined themselves as 'successfully' rehabilitated. The findings contributed to rehabilitation therapists' gaining an understanding of the unique client experiences of living with the disability resulting from spinal cord injury and the positive factors that contributed to their 'getting on with life'.

Ethnography

Ethnography originated in cultural anthropology and, as such, is traditionally associated with the exploration and description of "primitive" cultures by early twentieth century anthropologists such as Malinowski (1922). In the 1920s and 1930s the methodology was adapted by sociologists, such as Mead (1928), primarily located at the University of Chicago, with the aim of studying cultural groups, for example poor and marginalized groups within the larger United States society. In recent years, ethnography has been used to develop holistic descriptions and understanding of practice by other disciplines in education and health care. Within the health care context, it is not difficult to recognize cultural groups within different settings. Examples of these could be people who share common settings such as long-term care facilities, IVF clinics, rehabilitation centers, intensive care units and maternity wards, or groups of people who share a similar issue, such as those who have weight problems or who have survived childhood physical abuse.

The ethnographic theoretical tradition is based on the central assumption that 'knowledge of all cultures is valuable' (Spradley, 1979, p. 9). However, in recent years ethnography has diffused widely from its original intellectual source to other contexts of inquiry (Morse, 1994) and has been influenced by other theoretical perspectives, including phenomenology, symbolic interactionism, hermeneutics and feminism (Rice & Ezzy, 1999). In addition, a number of subtypes of ethnography have been developed, such as ethnomethodology (Francis & Hester, 2004). These influences represent a movement away from the search for cultural consensus, for the 'essential' features of a cultural group associated with traditional ethnographic research, and towards an increased interest in discernible behaviors and understandings connected with group cohesion and recognition of the differences or conflicts existing within social groups, for example power or access to health care services (Angrosino, 2005; Sharkey & Larsen, 2005). The sociological approach (Hammersley & Atkinson, 1995) has had the greatest influence on ethnographic research in health care and will be the primary focus of this discussion.

Congruent with the unstructured and flexible nature of ethnography, research usually starts with a broadly defined question that may change as the research progresses, and as the researcher responds to encounters and experiences in the field (Sharkey & Larsen, 2005). In a *focused ethnography*, the research design is predetermined and a detailed rationale for design decisions is provided, and the linkages between the research question or aim, data collection methods and analytic process are established. Such an approach may seem to contradict the flexible nature of ethnography but this more specific approach does seek to explore cultural understanding from the *insider* point of view. In health care, use of focused ethnography may be predicated on practical issues, such as feasibility, gaining access to informants and ethical review requirements (Morse & Field, 1995).

The aim of ethnography is to provide 'an insider perspective on everyday life through the researcher's engagement with people over time and explore human experience and social interaction as well as the meaning people apply to their experiences, that is, their symbolic world' (Sharkey & Larsen, 2005, p. 168). The intention is to develop a rich or *thick description* that interprets and facilitates a greater understanding of the experiences of people within the cultural group. As Creswell (1998) suggests, culture is 'an amorphous term', but in the context of ethnographic research it can be viewed as 'something the researcher attributes to the group [of interest]' (p. 59). The expression of this culture is embedded in the routine and mundane patterns of daily living and inferred from the words, actions, interactions and emotions of members of the group. *Participant observation* has been the primary method of ethnographic data generation. However, sociological ethnography tends to use multiple methods of collecting information in an effort to *triangulate* and test the validity of the information gathered (Angrosino, 2005). The methods used include all those associated with qualitative research. Participant observation continues to be characteristic of ethnography, but is frequently combined with other interactive methods, such as in-depth interviews, focus groups and life history accounts. These can also be supplemented by non-interactive or unobtrusive methods. Such methods draw social and cultural meanings from existing sources, such as medical records, meeting minutes, audiovisual records or photographs, and provide the 'story behind the story' (Rice & Ezzy, 1999, p. 166). These methods are described in more detail in Chapter 5.

The nature of ethnography is interpersonal. It requires researchers to *immerse* themselves in the culture of interest and to establish collaborative relationships with the informants. As a result, the concept of *reflexivity* (see Chapter 7 for a more detailed discussion of this concept) is of paramount importance at every phase of the research process. The researcher is the key instrument and the researcher's understanding, theoretical knowledge, insights and values are brought to bear on all aspects of the research process and need to be made explicit. This is achieved by rigorous and thorough documentation. These documents then become data for the study rather than a 'methodological problem' which is external to the research process and which needs to be resolved (Wallace, 2005, p. 76). The documentary evidence in ethnography takes the form of field notes and analytic memos or notes. These core ethnographic strategies are also commonly employed in other qualitative research approaches. *Field notes* are accounts describing experiences and observations the researcher has made while participating in an intense and involved manner (with the group members) (Rice & Ezzy, 1999). They are the primary data arising from ethnographic *fieldwork* and are integral to the participant observation method. Field notes represent the social reality of the group of interest, and also provide essential information about the researcher's perceptions, ongoing theoretical decisions and interpretations. Because of the central role of field notes in ethnographic research, they need to be rigorously and systematically recorded (see Chapter 6 for further discussion). *Analytic memos or notes*, as in grounded theory, are an integral part of the data analysis process. Through them, the researcher consistently reflects on emerging ideas and interpretations and the contribution that prior theoretical knowledge and *sensitizing concepts* make to the analytic process. Memo writing reinforces the flexible nature of ethnography by encouraging the researcher not only to seek answers but to ask critical questions of the informants and the data.

Traditionally, ethnographic researchers were not members of the culture or group to be studied. In such cases, researchers need to gain access to the setting or group and this is frequently a time-consuming process involving a number of political, ethical and legal issues. The role of *gatekeeper* is associated with these issues of gaining access. However, gatekeepers are rarely neutral and can have considerable influence on the researcher's relationship with the group members, the informants accessed and the direction the research takes. These influences need to be critically monitored if a gatekeeper is involved. Sharkey & Larsen (2005) warn that 'using a gatekeeper indicates a social alliance and the status and role of the gatekeeper is likely to be "carried" by the researcher in the research setting at least initially' (p. 173). These issues can be avoided if the researcher is an *insider*, that is, a member of the group. This is frequently the situation in health care research; however, the dual role of practitioner and researcher can be problematic. Research that entails studying members of the researcher's own professional group or colleagues, or working with participants who have been clients, requires a careful and ongoing negotiation and clarification of the difference between the researcher role and the professional or therapeutic roles. Ethnographic researchers frequently identify and work with *key informants* to produce an accurate description of the culture (Rice & Ezzy, 1999). These are individuals who are able to articulate their experience of the culture clearly and provide in-depth information, and who are chosen for their cultural competence rather than their representativeness (see Chapter 5).

In summary, ethnography has a long history of contributing to the understanding of the complexities of social interaction within a group or culture. Used in health care, an ethnographic approach utilizes multiple methods of data generation most of which require the researcher to engage in intense interaction with members of the group of interest, and to *immerse* themselves over a prolonged period of time. Some concepts are particularly associated with the ethnographic tradition, for example participant observation, gatekeepers, key informants, the emic or insider perspective and reflexivity, although most of these are now applied in other qualitative research approaches. The end product of ethnography is a rich interpretation of the culture or a specific cultural phenomenon of interest and this usually takes the form of narrative account. In this way, the ethnographic researcher not only conducts an ethnography but also writes an ethnography. An example of an ethnographic study is provided by Pellatt (2004) who conducted a *ethnographic* study, using semi-structured interviews and participant observation, to explore and describe patients' and professionals' experiences of patient participation in team decision-making. Townsend *et al.* (2003) describe an ethnographic study they conducted to explore the influence and impact of the institutional context on the delivery of mental health occupational therapy services, and the detailed account makes fascinating reading for practitioners all too familiar with the disempowering and constraining nature of institutional structures.

Participatory action research (PAR)

Participatory action research began with social psychologist Lewin's (1948) work with community action groups in the United States and, more recently, has been developed by educators, such as Freire (1970) and Fals-Borda (1988), in the context of social movements in the developing world (Kemmis & McTaggert, 2005). It has been widely adopted in education, particularly in exploring teaching and learning practice (McNiff & Whitehead, 2006). Action research has a complex history and there is a continuing debate about what counts as action research. However, PAR is emerging as the most widely practiced action approach in health care (Letts, 2003).

The key concepts that define PAR are participation and *conscientization*, Freire's (1970) term for 'a process of self-awareness through collective self-inquiry and reflection' (Fals-Borda & Rahman, 1991, p. 16). Reason (1998) describes PAR as a strategy, rather than a methodology, which focuses primarily on ontological concerns. Reason (1998) articulates the main aims of PAR as the production of 'knowledge and action directly useful to a group of people – through research, adult education, and sociopolitical action' and the empowerment of 'people at a second and deeper level though the process of constructing and using their own knowledge' (p. 269). The unique characteristics of PAR are outlined in Reason & Bradbury's (2001) definition of PAR as:

> A participatory, democratic process concerned with developing practical knowing in the pursuit of worthwhile human purposes, grounded in a participatory worldview that we believe is emerging at this historical moment. It seeks to bring together action and reflection, theory and practice, in participation with others, in the pursuit of practical solutions to issues of pressing concern to people, and generally the flourishing of individual persons and their communities (p. 1).

The underlying principles of PAR – democratic action, participation, empowerment and respect – are clearly congruent with the concepts of client-centered practice, advocacy and occupation in occupational therapy (Letts, 2003) and also align with recent government directives, for example 'expert' patient initiatives (Department of Health, 2001, 2005). Kemmis & McTaggert (2005) identify three characteristics often used to distinguish PAR from other research approaches: 'shared ownership of research projects, community-based analysis of social problems, and an orientation toward community action' (p. 560).

Participatory action research is theoretically most closely aligned with qualitative methodologies, such as critical ethnography, and is generally described as a form of qualitative research (Reason, 1998). However, PAR is a systematic process of inquiry that can utilize both qualitative and quantitative methods (Stringer & Genat, 2004). One of the major strengths of PAR is its emergent quality – its ability to enable researchers to tentatively state the problem, then refine and reframe the study by continuing iterations of a cyclical model of research. This model is typically presented as a spiral helix indicating that the four phases – planning, acting, observing and reflecting – of research are repeated over time (Stringer & Genat, 2004). This cyclical process continues until an effective solution to the problem has been attained. A more complex model of action research has been developed by Stringer & Genat (2004) that may prove useful for those working in conjunction with university or professional environments. It provides the more detailed outline of the research design, activities and methods that may be required in developing research proposals and gaining ethical approval. The methods used to collect data in PAR studies are most commonly those associated with qualitative methodologies, for example in-depth interviews, observation, focus groups and reviewing records and other documentation. However, depending on the research purpose, quantitative methods, such as the use of outcome measures and questionnaires, can be appropriate. A key feature of PAR, in addressing the complex and multidimensional issues in health care service delivery and practice, is the developmental nature of the process, that is, initial inquiries are focused on tangible and achievable objectives. As these objectives are resolved, new dimensions of the problem are identified and investigated through continuous iterations of the cyclical process.

A major purpose of PAR is 'to bring people together in a dialogic and productive relationship, enabling the development of a sense of community through the sharing of perspectives, the negotiation of meaning, and the development of collaboratively produced activities, programs and projects' (Stringer & Genat, 2004, p. 9). It focuses on achieving positive social change and in order to fulfill this purpose a re-conceptualization of the roles of the external researcher and participants in the PAR process is required. The role of the researcher has traditionally been to determine the research agenda, and to design and implement the study. The assumption is that the researcher possesses the knowledge, gained from training and experience, needed to direct the research process.

The roles in PAR are, however, not as easy to define. It is often acknowledged that PAR projects would not be initiated, gain funding, or be implemented without the attention of an 'outside' researcher (Letts, 2003), but there are challenges associated with this leadership or facilitation role. In PAR, the researcher acts more like a consultant who brings a particular skill set to integrate with those skills brought to the project by other participants. This individual, however, cannot simply focus on the 'method' of action research but needs to be committed to participate in the personal and social changes in practice that have brought the participants together (Kemmis & McTaggert, 2005). If control within the process is assigned to one participant more than others then the collaborative and democratic nature of PAR is undermined. In addition, when academics participate in PAR research there is a risk that the research will be driven by the demands of the organization rather than the researchers (Letts, 2003). Generally, both researcher and participants are *stakeholders* in the purpose and process, that is, they have a stake in the research and its outcome because they are affected by the issue in question and have an influence on events related to the issue (Stringer & Genat, 2004). In PAR, the ideal is 'when all participants become researchers in their own right, gaining the skills and insights that enable them to systematically investigate issues in their own lives' (Stringer & Genat, 2004, p. 10).

In summary, in PAR the motivation to act is to resolve a common problem. It means working and negotiating with people at all stages of the process. The approach is ongoing, open-ended, developmental and dynamic, and can be represented as a cyclical process involving the use of a diversity of data collection and analysis methods (McNiff & Whitehead, 2006). PAR is 'directed deliberately toward discovering, investigating, and attaining intersubjective agreement, mutual understanding and unforced consensus about [how to proceed in the process]' (Kemmis & McTaggert, 2005, p. 578). Atwal (2002) and Law (2004) provide two examples of PAR studies conducted by occupational therapists. Atwal (2002) describes an action research study that took place in an inner-city London teaching hospital on an acute orthopedic ward, over a seven-month period. The aim of the study was to enhance interprofessional team functioning by developing and implementing a new interprofessional discharge model for patients with a fractured neck of femur. Law (2004) worked with parents of children with physical disabilities, using a PAR research design, to identify environmental situations that presented challenges for their children. Towards the end of the project the parents organized themselves into a support and advocacy group and pursued a number of policy recommendations with local government agencies.

The methodological debate

Qualitative scholars and theorists (for example Thorne, 1997; Avis, 2003) continue to vigorously debate the need and use of methodological theory in qualitative research. They are concerned that the methodological detail required of researchers, particularly those with less experience, is becoming excessive and they call instead for a greater understanding of the essential epistemological distinctions between interpretivist and positivist research. However, a lack of understanding is frequently evident in published study reports, where the authors use inappropriate language in describing their research design, for example subjects instead of participants or informants, randomization instead of purposive sampling and generalizability instead of transferability. In our experience the application of an appropriate methodological theory to the research process contributes to a coherent qualitative research design and rigorous analysis process. As Avis (2003) points out, 'methodological justification concerns the rationale given for the characteristic techniques used in the production of empirical evidence within a particular research tradition' (p. 1003). Frequently, researchers simply describe a specific method, such as focus group, and use qualitative terminology, such as constant comparison method or content analysis, with no evidence of the theoretical context or methodological grounding of the terms. Researchers have the responsibility of creating 'methodologically convincing stories' (Miller & Crabtree, 2005, p. 626) by providing a cogent rationale for their proposed research study based on an in-depth understanding of a methodological approach. Such understanding is achieved by critically reflecting on the social roles and values of the research team, the social processes of generating evidence, the relationship of theory to practice, and the purpose of the research and the impact on those "being studied".

In this chapter, we have introduced four methodologies or theoretical approaches – grounded theory, phenomenology, ethnography and participatory action research – that we think have significant relevance to investigating issues related to rehabilitation practice. In the next chapter we will discuss the practicalities of involving participants in qualitative studies and review a number of data collection methods.

References

Angrosino, M.V. (2005) Recontextualizing observation: ethnography, pedagogy, and the prospects for a progressive political agenda. In: N.K. Denzin & Y.S. Lincoln (eds), *The Sage Handbook of Qualitative Research* (3rd edn, pp. 729–745). Thousand Oaks, Calif., Sage.

Atwal, A. (2002) Getting evidence into practice: the challenges and successes of action research. *British Journal of Occupational Therapy*, 65 (7), 335–341.

Avis, M. (2003) Do we need methodological theory to do qualitative research? *Qualitative Health Research*, 13 (7), 995–1004.

Benner, P. (1994) *Interpretive Phenomenology: Embodiment, Caring, and Ethics in Health and Illness*. Thousand Oaks, Calif., Sage.

Bluff, R. (2005) Grounded theory: the methodology. In: I. Holloway (ed.), *Qualitative Research in Health Care* (pp. 147–167). Oxford, Blackwell.

Carpenter, C. (1994) The experience of spinal cord injury: the individual's perspective – implications for rehabilitation practice. *Physical Therapy*, 74 (7), 614–629.

Charmaz, K. (2000) Grounded theory: objectivist and constructivist methods. In: N.K. Denzin & Y.S. Lincoln (eds), *Handbook of Qualitative Research* (2nd edn, pp. 509–535). Thousand Oaks, Calif., Sage.

Charmaz, K. (2005) Grounded theory in the twenty-first century: applications for advancing social justice studies. In: N.K. Denzin & Y.S. Lincoln (eds), *The Sage Handbook of Qualitative Research* (3rd edn, pp. 507–526). Thousand Oaks, Calif., Sage.

Creswell, J.W. (1998) *Qualitative Inquiry and Research Design: Choosing Among Five Traditions.* Thousand Oaks, Calif., Sage.

Denzin, N.K. & Lincoln, Y.S. (2005) Introduction: the discipline and practice of qualitative research. In: N.K. Denzin & Y.S. Lincoln (eds), *The Sage Handbook of Qualitative Research* (3rd edn, pp. 1–32). Thousand Oaks, Calif., Sage.

Department of Health (2001) *The Expert Patient: a New Approach to Chronic Disease Management for the Twenty-first Century.* London, Department of Health.

Department of Health (2005) *Creating a Patient-led NHS: Delivering the NHS Improvement Plan.* London, Department of Health.

Fals-Borda, O. (1988) *Knowledge and People's Power: Lessons with Peasants in Nicaragua, Mexico and Columbia.* New Delhi, Indian Social Institute.

Fals-Borda, O. & Rahman, M.A. (eds) (1991) *Action and Knowledge: Breaking the Monopoly with Participatory Action Research.* New York, The Apex Press.

Finlay, L. (1999) Applying phenomenology in research: problems, principles and practice. *British Journal of Occupational Therapy*, 62 (7), 299–306.

Francis, D. & Hester, S. (2004) *An Invitation to Ethnomethodology: Language, Society and Interaction.* London, Sage.

Freire, P. (1970) *Pedagogy of the Oppressed.* New York, Herder & Herder.

Giorgi, A. (1985) *A Sketch of a Psychological Phenomenological Method.* Pittsburgh, Duquesne University.

Giorgi, A. (1997) The theory, practice and evaluation of the phenomenological method as a qualitative research procedure. *Journal of Phenomenological Psychology*, 28 (2), 235–260.

Giorgi, A. & Giorgi, B. (2003a) Phenomenology. In: J.A. Smith (ed.), *Qualitative Psychology: a Practical Guide to Research Methods* (pp. 25–50). Thousand Oaks, Calif., Sage.

Giorgi, A. & Giorgi, B. (2003b) The descriptive phenomenological psychological method. In: P.M. Camic, J.E. Rhodes & L. Yardley (eds), *Qualitative Research in Psychology: Expanding Perspectives in Methodology and Design* (pp. 243–273). Washington, DC, American Psychological Association.

Glaser, B.G. (1992) *Basics of Grounded Theory Analysis: Emergence vs Forced.* Mill Valley, Calif., Sociology Press.

Glaser, B.G. & Strauss, A.L. (1967) *The Discovery of Grounded Theory: Strategies for Qualitative Research.* Chicago, Aldine.

Glaser, B.G. & Strauss, A.L. (1968) *Time for Dying.* Chicago, Aldine.

Hammersley, M. & Atkinson, P. (1995) *Ethnography: Principles in Practice* (2nd edn). London, Routledge.

Kemmis, S. & McTaggert, R. (2005) Participatory action research: communicative action and the public sphere. In: N.K. Denzin & Y.S. Lincoln (eds), *The Sage Handbook of Qualitative Research*, (3rd edn, pp. 559–603). Thousand Oaks, Calif., Sage.

Law, M. (2004) Building knowledge through participatory research. In: K.W. Hammell & C. Carpenter (eds), *Qualitative Research in Evidence-based Rehabilitation* (pp. 40–50). Edinburgh, Churchill Livingstone.

Letts, L. (2003) Occupational therapy and participatory research: a partnership worth pursuing. *American Journal of Occupational Therapy, 57* (1), 77–87.

Lewin, K. (1948) *Resolving Social Conflicts; Selected Papers on Group Dynamics.* Gertrude W. Lewin (ed.). New York, Harper & Row.

McNiff, J. & Whitehead, J. (2006) *All You Need to Know About Action Research.* Thousand Oaks, Calif., Sage.

Malinowski, B. (1922) *Argonauts of the Western Pacific.* London, Routledge & Kegan Paul.

Mead, M. (1928) *Coming of Age in Samoa.* New York, William Morrow.

Merleau-Ponty, M. (1962) *The Phenomenology of Perception.* Trans by C. Smith. London, Routledge & Kegan Paul.

Miller, W.L. & Crabtree, B.F. (2005) Clinical research. In: N.K. Denzin & Y.S. Lincoln (eds), *The Sage Handbook of Qualitative Research* (3rd edn, pp. 605–639). Thousand Oaks, Calif., Sage.

Morse, J.M. (ed.) (1994) *Critical Issues in Qualitative Research Methods.* Thousand Oaks, Calif., Sage.

Morse, J.M. (1995) The significance of data saturation. *Qualitative Health Research, 5,* 147–149.

Morse, J.M. & Field, P.A. (1995) *Qualitative Research Methods for Health Professionals.* Thousand Oaks, Calif., Sage.

Moustakas, C. (1994) *Phenomenological Research Methods.* Thousand Oaks, Calif., Sage.

Pellatt, G.C. (2004) Patient-professional partnership in spinal cord injury rehabilitation rehabilitation. *British Journal of Nursing,* 13(16), 948–953.

Rapport, F. (2005) Hermeneutic phenomenology: the science of interpretation of texts. In: I. Holloway (ed.), *Qualitative Research in Health Care* (pp. 125–146). Oxford, Blackwell.

Reason, P. (1998) Three approaches to participative inquiry. In: N.K. Denzin & Y.S. Lincoln (eds), *Strategies of Qualitative Inquiry* (pp. 261–291). Thousand Oaks, Calif., Sage.

Reason, P. & Bradbury, H. (eds) (2001) *Handbook of Action Research: Participative Inquiry and Practice.* London, Sage.

Rice, L.P. & Ezzy, D. (1999) *Qualitative Research Methods.* Oxford, Oxford University Press.

Rose, L., Mallinson, R.K. & Walton-Moss, B. (2002) A grounded theory of families responding to mental illness. *Western Journal of Nursing Research, 24* (5), 516–536.

Schachter, C., Stalker, C. & Teram, E. (1999) Toward sensitive practice: issues for physical therapists working with survivors of childhood abuse. *Physical Therapy, 79* (3), 248–261.

Schachter, C., Stalker, C. & Teram, E. (2001) *Handbook on Sensitive Practice for Health Professionals: Lessons from Women Survivors of Childhood Sexual Abuse.* Ottawa, Health Canada.

Schutz, A. (1972) *The Phenomenology of the Social World.* Trans by G. Walsh & F. Lehnert. London, Heinemann.

Sharkey, S. & Larsen, J.A. (2005) Ethnographic exploration: participation and meaning in everyday life. In: I. Holloway (ed.), *Qualitative Research in Health Care* (pp. 168–190). Oxford, Blackwell.

Smith, J.A. (2003) *Qualitative Psychology: a Practical Guide to Research Methods.* London, Sage.

Spradley, J.P. (1979) *The Ethnographic Interview*. New York, Holt, Rinehart & Winston.

Strauss, A.L. & Corbin, J. (1990) *Basics of Qualitative Research: Grounded Theory Procedures and Techniques*. Newbury Park, Calif., Sage.

Strauss, A.L. & Corbin, J. (1994) Grounded theory methodology: an overview. In: N.K. Denzin & Y.S. Lincoln (eds), *Handbook of Qualitative Research* (pp. 273–285). Thousand Oaks, Calif., Sage.

Strauss, A.L. & Corbin, J. (1998) *Basics of Qualitative Research: Techniques and Procedures for Developing Grounded Theory*. Thousand Oaks, Calif., Sage.

Stringer, E. & Genat, W.J. (2004) *Action Research in Health*. Peer Saddle River, NJ, Pearson/Merrill Prentice Hall.

Thorne, S. (1997) Phenomenological positivism and other problematic trends in health science research. *Qualitative Health Research*, 7 (2), 287–293.

Todres, L. (2005) Clarifying the life-world: descriptive phenomenology. In: I. Holloway (ed.), *Qualitative Research in Health Care* (pp. 104–124). Oxford, Blackwell.

Townsend, E., Langille, L. & Ripley, D. (2003) Professional tensions in client-centered practice: using institutional ethnography to generate understanding and transformation. *American Journal of Occupational Therapy*, 57 (1), 17–28.

van Manen, M. (1990) *Researched Experience: Human Science for an Action Sensitive Pedagogy*. London, Ont., Althouse.

van Manen, M. (1997) From meaning to method. *Qualitative Health Research*, 7 (3), 345–369.

Wallace, S. (2005) Observing method: recognizing the significance of belief, discipline, position and documentation in observational studies. In: I. Holloway (ed.), *Qualitative Research in Health Care* (pp. 71–89). Oxford, Blackwell.

Chapter 5
INVOLVING PARTICIPANTS AND DATA COLLECTION METHODS

Introduction

In this chapter, we begin to address the central practical issues of conducting a qualitative research study: recruitment of participants, data collection and the desirability of conducting a pilot study. We will specifically discuss the sampling strategies and methods of data collection: in-depth interviews, focus groups, participant observation, consensus and 'unobtrusive' approaches. It is at this stage that researchers feel they are actually doing research. It can be tempting to move directly to choosing a method, involving participants and collecting data, without creating 'methodologically convincing stories' (Miller & Crabtree, 2005, p. 626) that require us, as researchers, to justify the practical and ethical decisions we make. Sampling is another term that has been primarily associated with quantitative research, where it is a process of selecting people or organizations from a population of interest so that by studying the sample researchers can generalize the research results. In qualitative research, sampling strategies are guided more by the desire to recruit participants who can contribute their understanding or experience of the phenomena of interest than an interest in the generalizability of the findings. Because the data collection methods in qualitative research entail a direct and sometimes prolonged interaction between the researcher and participants, and the phenomena being investigated may be of a sensitive nature, every effort must be made to ensure that the recruitment process is ethical (see Chapter 3).

Sampling strategies in qualitative research

Purposive sampling

Purposive sampling strategies are primarily used in qualitative research and are also referred to as theoretical, non-probability or purposeful sampling. In this book we will use the terms *purposive or theoretical sampling*. The latter term was initially introduced in relation to grounded theory by Glaser & Strauss (1967) and later revised by Strauss & Corbin (1990). However, many qualitative researchers use the terms theoretical and purposive sampling interchangeably, without necessarily adhering to the precise techniques recommended by these authors (Mason,

2002). Purposive sampling can be defined as the selection of individuals, groups of individuals or institutions based on specific purposes associated with addressing the research study's questions or aim (Teddlie & Yu, 2007). It involves deliberately selecting particular settings, persons, or events for the important information they can provide that cannot be acquired as effectively through other means.

There are three broad purposive sampling approaches based on the specific purpose or aim of the research:

1. *Sampling to achieve representativeness or comparability* with the aim of increasing or facilitating *transferability* of the findings. A more detailed discussion of transferability can be found in Chapter 9. Teddlie & Yu (2007), using a number of different sources, identified six types of purposive sampling procedures, which focus on finding representative or typical instances of a particular topic or phenomenon of interest, or comparing it across different participants or situations. These types are described as *typical case, extreme* or *deviant case* (also called *outlier sampling), intensity, maximum variation, homogeneous* and *reputational sampling*. These six descriptors are fairly self-evident, for example extreme or deviant case sampling 'involves selecting those cases that are the most outstanding successes or failures related to the topic of interest' (Teddlie & Yu, 2007, p. 81). Researchers often simply describe their sampling approach as purposive, but identifying the type of strategy more definitively contributes to the coherence of the study design decisions. Comparisons or contrasts of participants or cases are integral to the qualitative data analysis process, in particular the constant comparative approach in grounded theory (Glaser & Strauss, 1967; Mason, 2002).

2. *Sampling special or unique cases* has traditionally been the focus of qualitative research in anthropology and sociology. Stake (2000) suggests that as a form of research, a *case study* is defined by the intrinsic interest in individual cases rather than the overall issues or the methods of inquiry. In his view 'case study is not a methodological choice but a choice of what is to be studied' (p. 435) and, therefore, identification or sampling of the cases is of paramount importance. In quantitative research, the case study approach focuses on individual persons and the collection of 'comparable data points' from each case (Miles & Huberman, 1994, p. 29). A qualitative 'case' may be an individual person, but can also be defined more broadly as a text, role, group, organization, program or culture. The researcher makes sampling decisions within the case, such as activities, observable behaviors, times, locations and significant others (Ritchie, 2001). The evidence from multiple cases is often considered more compelling and the overall study design more robust (Yin, 2003). Multiple-case sampling adds to the trustworthiness or credibility of the findings and each case should serve a specific purpose within the overall scope of the inquiry (Yin, 2003). Each case contributes to an understanding of the phenomenon of interest and to the development of an emerging theoretical framework. Use of a *sampling frame* is recommended in multiple-case qualitative research (Miles & Huberman, 1994; Mason, 2002; Yin, 2003). A sampling

frame is a resource from which a researcher can select a smaller sample, for example membership of a professional or disability advocacy organization, or client/patient lists of a specific health care program. Such a resource may facilitate access to the specific sample needed for the study but it may also constrain the nature and diversity of the information acquired. A sampling frame may not be available and in this situation a sequential sampling approach, such as snowball sampling, can be employed.

3. *Sequential sampling* aims to access a relevant range of contexts or phenomena, for example experiences, characteristics, processes, types, cases or examples, which will enable the researcher to make comparisons and build a defendable, well-founded argument or theory (Mason, 2002). The sample is designed to reflect, but not represent directly, the larger group or context. Three types of purposive sampling techniques are defined as sequential: theoretical, opportunistic and snowball sampling. *Theoretical sampling* is concerned with constructing a sample, often at different stages of the data collection and analysis process, which is meaningful because it builds in certain characteristics or criteria that contribute to the development and testing of an emerging theory or argument (Mason, 2002). In using an *opportunistic sampling* strategy, the researcher, guided by the research purpose and conceptual framework, selects a suitable sample simply as the opportunity presents itself. *Snowball sampling* is related to opportunistic sampling in that the researcher initially identifies one or two informants with knowledge or experience of the topic of interest and asks them if they know others who might meet the sampling requirement and who might be interested in being involved in the study. In this way successive participants are involved in the study and a snowball effect is created.

Convenience sampling

Convenience sampling involves accessing people who are conveniently available and willing to participate in a study, and two types have been described: *captive* (for example students in a class) and *volunteer* (for example colleagues in a physiotherapy department). This sampling strategy can be differentiated from purposive sampling approaches as it lacks the explicit use of conceptual frameworks or theoretical focus characteristic of the latter and it is not commonly used in qualitative research.

In summary, theoretical or purposive sampling can be criticized for being vague and overly influenced by the researcher. It is therefore important to demonstrate a logical, systematic and ethical approach to recruiting participants and to provide a detailed description of the sampling strategies used.

Determining sample size

Decisions about sample size in qualitative research can be difficult both to make and to defend when asked questions like, 'Why such a small number?' 'How do you know the sample will be representative?' and 'How are you going to avoid bias?' Questions like this represent the assumptions of representativeness, normal distribution and generalizability that underpin quantitative and survey approaches. An inability to defend sampling strategies and sample size decisions in qualitative research often reflects a lack of understanding of the different set of characteristics that underpin qualitative research discussed in Chapter 2. It is all too easy to slide back into statistical or probability logic and wrongly apply terms like 'representative' and 'bias' to a qualitative study design. For example, it would be illogical to view one 55-year-old informant in a study as representative of all 55-year-olds (Mason, 2002), or researcher 'bias' as something to be accounted for and controlled. Qualitative researchers actively seek to recruit participants who can represent well and have experience of the phenomenon of interest. The sampling strategies are of necessity *biased* (Morse, 1998). The key is to focus the participant selection strategically and meaningfully, rather than to create a representative sample (Mason, 2002).

The key question to ask when making sampling decisions is whether the sample provides access to enough data, and with the right focus, to enable the research question or purpose to be thoroughly addressed (Mason, 2002). The sample size and range of participants are intended to generate sufficient data to explore processes, similarities and differences, to develop theory and descriptions that take into account specific contexts, rather than to make statistical comparisons or infer causal relationships. In qualitative research there is no set formula for determining the sample size (Morse, 1998). *Data saturation* is a concept associated with grounded theory (see Chapter 4) that has been more broadly adopted by qualitative researchers as a means of justifying participant recruitment decisions and ending the data collection process. Saturation is presumed to have occurred when little or no new information about the topic of interest is being acquired and new data fits into the categories already developed in the data analysis process.

There are a number of other factors to consider in making sample size decisions, such as the scope of the study, the nature of the topic, the amount of useful information obtained from each participant or source (for example medical records), and the methodology and methods used in the study design (Morse, 2000). The broader the scope of the research question, the more participants or data sources will be needed, the more data will be generated and the longer it will take to reach data saturation. If the topic is fairly straightforward and non-controversial, the data are more easily obtained and fewer participants are needed. However, if the topic is more sensitive and difficult for the participants to talk about or 'difficult to grab', then the number of participants may need to be increased (Morse, 2000, p. 4). The quality and comprehensiveness of the data acquired varies with different participants or sources of information. Some participants have more experience with the topic of interest, are able to reflect deeply on their experiences, are less distracted and more focused on the topic of interest, or are simply more articulate (Morse, 2000). The greater the quality of data acquired from each source, the smaller the sample size required.

The research design, that is the methodological approach and associated methods of data collection, can influence the sampling strategy and sample size. *Theoretical sampling* is a defining concept of grounded theory and pivotal to the goal of theory development (Charmaz, 2000). As researchers engage in the zigzag process of data collection and analysis, described in Chapter 4, they use theoretical sampling to develop emerging categories and to refine ideas. By identifying and selecting participants with specific experiences and knowledge at different stages of the data analysis process, emerging theoretical concepts and relationships can be confirmed or discarded, gaps identified and constructs explained. Theory development is no lightweight endeavor and consequently grounded theory usually requires a bigger sample size than other methodological approaches; for example, Schachter *et al.* (1999) continued to conduct in-depth interviews with women who were survivors of childhood abuse until they felt data saturation had been reached. Twenty-seven women were ultimately recruited and a further eight were involved in the second phase, during which the conceptual framework of sensitive practice was critiqued and applied in developing guidelines for sensitive physical therapy practice.

In contrast, a phenomenological approach focuses on determining the *essence* of an individual's experience or phenomenon. This is usually achieved by recruiting a small number of participants using a rigorous purposive sampling strategy and conducting one to three in-depth interviews with each participant. Participant recruitment is ended when the information gained from the interviews becomes repetitive; for example, Carpenter (1994) conducted long in-depth, semi-structured interviews with ten participants before ending data collection.

In ethnography, triangulation of the data obtained about the culture or group of interest is an essential feature of the study design. Data resulting from a variety of data collection methods are frequently combined. The choice of sampling strategies and sample size for each method depends on the scope and nature of the study but the overall aim is to provide a comprehensive description of group interaction and experiences.

Participatory action research starts from a different premise than the other methodologies described. It focuses on the involvement of stakeholders in all phases of the research process with the aim of achieving change in practice. At different phases, the stakeholders can assume the role of participant or researcher and both qualitative and quantitative methods of data collection can be utilized. As a result, participant recruitment decisions arise from guidelines associated with specific methods, such as focus groups or application of an outcome measurement tool.

In the next section, we will briefly discuss the methods most commonly used in qualitative research, that is, in-depth interviews, focus groups, participant observation, consensus and 'unobtrusive' approaches. The choice of data collection method is guided by the nature of the research question and the methodological choice and these linkages will be discussed in relation to each method described.

Data collection methods

Qualitative interviews

The interview is probably the most commonly employed data collection method in qualitative research (Fontana & Frey, 2000). Qualitative interviews are most frequently described as being on a continuum with unstructured interviews at one end and structured at the other. Mason (2002) makes a cogent argument against the use of these descriptors. In her opinion, 'the term "unstructured" interviewing is a misnomer because no research interview can be completely lacking some form of structure' (p. 62). Conversely, the inclusion of open-ended 'qualitative' questions in a structured interview, for example a questionnaire in survey research, does *not* constitute qualitative interviewing. The term 'semi-structured', occupying the middle ground on this continuum, like 'structured', suggests that an emphasis is placed on the process of administering questions and obtaining the desired response rather than the interpretive focus and flexibility more characteristic of qualitative interviewing. The terms associated with qualitative interviewing are confusing and for the sake of clarity we will use the terms *focused interview* or *in-depth interview* to describe qualitative interviewing.

We live in an interview society where the interview as a means of data gathering has become a common inquiry tool. Health care professionals routinely "take histories" and conduct interviews with patients as an integral part of their clinical practice and there is a danger that the substantial differences between clinical and qualitative interviewing may not be recognized (Britten, 2000). In-depth interviewing for the purposes of research can appear 'deceptively simple' (Sandelowski, 2002, p. 105) and researchers might be tempted to choose to interview without critically exploring the theoretical rationale behind their choices or ensuring coherence of the research design (Sandelowski, 2002; Rubin & Rubin, 2005; Taylor, 2005).

The choice of qualitative interviewing is supported and justified by the interpretive and constructivist theoretical frameworks that were discussed in Chapter 2. These important theoretical perspectives emphasize that the meanings that people attribute to an experience or situation are what is important. Further, these meanings are constructed and reconstructed through interaction, relationship and in response to different contexts. *In-depth interviews* focus on 'the *hows* of people's lives (the constructive work involved in producing order in everyday life) as well as the traditional *whats* (the activities of everyday life)' (Fontana & Frey, 2000, p. 646). The overall purpose or aim of qualitative interviewing as suggested by Jones (cited by Taylor, 2005, p. 41) clearly reflects these theoretical perspectives:

> To understand other people's constructions of reality we would do well to ask them (rather than assume we know merely by observing their overt behavior) and to ask them in such a way that they can tell us on their own terms (rather than those imposed rigidly and *a priori* by ourselves) and in a depth which

addresses the rich context that is the substance of their meanings (rather than through isolated segments squeezed into a few lines on a paper).

The in-depth interview method of data collection is commonly used in rehabilitation studies (for example Maclean *et al.*, 2000; Marquis & Jackson, 2000; Ford *et al.*, 2002 Scheer *et al.*, 2003; Blank, 2004; Lund & Nygaard, 2004). The authors usually define their approach as being qualitative; however, very few justify their choice of the qualitative paradigm or identify the specific methodological framework of their study. In-depth interviews are a method of generating data that is used across different methodological approaches. In grounded theory, qualitative interviewing is used at all stages of data collection. Early in the process, when the aim is to understand the breadth and depth of the topic of interest, interviewing will be in-depth and loosely structured. As the study progresses, and concepts and theories begin to emerge and need to be explored in depth or validated, the interviews will become more focused. In phenomenology, where the aim is to understand the meaning individuals attribute to their lived experience, interviews are the primary data collection method. Interviewers attempt to *bracket* their preconceptions and assumptions and to be non-directive during the interview. They generally begin with broad opening questions and, as the interview progresses, probe and reflect their understanding back to the interviewee to ensure a full exploration of the experience is achieved. In ethnography, where the aim is to explore cultural meanings or processes, interviews are usually conducted to support or build on data obtained through participant observation. These interviews may take the form of informal conversations with key informants or be focused on asking members of the culture or group to explain observed behaviors or interactions. In health care, researchers may engage in focused ethnographies (Morse & Field, 1995) in which *ethnographic interviewing* is the primary data collection method (for example Carpenter, 2004; Bourke-Taylor & Hudson, 2005). In such studies, several interviews take place over a prolonged period of time, for example six months, and data are also gathered from other sources, such as videos, photographs and documents. In participatory action research (PAR), which is characterized by continuing iterations of a cyclical model (Stringer & Genat, 2004), qualitative interviewing may be chosen as the method consistent with the purpose of the research at any given stage of the process.

The flexibility and adaptability of qualitative interviewing is often characterized as a *purposeful conversation* or, as Rubin & Rubin (2005) describe it, responsive interviewing. While such interviews are most commonly conducted in face-to-face settings, they can also be carried out over the telephone, or via the Internet (see Chapter 10 for a more in-depth discussion). They can involve a single interview of 30 minutes or longer with each participant, or a series of lengthy interviews over a prolonged period of time. However, most studies in health care seem to consist of single interviews of approximately 90 minutes. Regardless of the type of qualitative interviewing, the importance of detailed and rigorous planning and the development of a specific set of skills should not be underestimated (Mason, 2002).

The art of qualitative interviewing is complex, creative and active, and is central to the role of *researcher as research instrument*. Qualitative interviewers have to be prepared to think on their feet, and make on-the-spot decisions about the content and sequence of the interview as it progresses in ways that are consistent with the research purpose. 'They need to ensure that the interview interaction actually does generate relevant data, which means simultaneously orchestrating the intellectual and social dynamics of the situation' (Mason, 2002, p. 67). The flexible nature of qualitative interviewing requires that interviewers, prior to engaging with participants, need to reflect on their interviewing style, how to be an active listener, decide on the breadth and scope of the questions and anticipate the need for prompts or probing questions. Researchers develop different styles compatible with their own personalities, such as encouraging while minimizing their own involvement, challenging, non-confrontational, or relationship building (Rubin & Rubin, 2005). During the interview, interviewers need to remember what the participants have said, achieve a balance between talking and listening, observe verbal and non-verbal cues and be responsive to the participant's reactions, maintain the flow of the interview and manage the practicalities of the interview process (Mason, 2002).

Analysis of the techniques used by effective interviewers reveals how they consistently use open-ended rather than leading or forced response questions and avoid multiple or double-barrelled questions, rarely use technical language or ask questions that appear to test knowledge, and ask probing questions that enable participants to describe their experiences more fully. Patton (2002) advocates considering several types of questions when planning a qualitative interview – behavioral, experiential, opinions or values, feelings or emotions, sensory and background – but stresses that each type of question needs to be consistent with the nature and purpose of the research. Rubin & Rubin (2005) identify some useful types of probes or prompts:

- Elaboration probes focused on encouraging the participant to provide more detail: 'Can you tell me a bit more about that?'
- Continuation probes encourage the participant to keep talking: 'What happened then?' 'How did that work out over time?' 'Have you experienced the same thing since?'
- Clarification probes aim to resolve confusion or uncertainty: 'I'm not sure I understand what you mean by that.' These can also involve restatement or paraphrasing of something that the participant has said, or the interviewer can reflect back what they understood was said for confirmation.
- Attention probes indicate that the interviewer is giving the participant their full attention: 'That's really interesting.'
- Contrast probes give the participant something to contradict or encourage them to provide more explanation: 'Are you suggesting a particular reason why that happened?' (p. 352)

Usually, the person who conducts the interview also manages the practicalities of the interview process. This includes deciding on a sampling strategy, making the initial contact with potential participants and ensuring that they are fully informed. Each interview may require a letter of introduction, a personal introduction, phone calls to schedule an interview and arrange a location, travel arrangements for the participant, an additional phone call to confirm the interview, arranging additional interviews if required and a thank you letter to the participant (Rice & Ezzy, 1999). In addition, during the interview the interviewer will need to record the interview either by audiotaping or by taking detailed notes or both. Tape recording the interview has advantages in that a complete record is made of the interview that does not rely on the interviewer's note-taking dexterity. It leaves the interviewer free to establish an authentic presence with the participant by making appropriate eye contact, developing useful questions and paying attention through actively listening. However, some participants do not wish to be taped and the equipment may malfunction. We have found it useful to make notes immediately after the interview, in which we have detailed any important insights gained from our interaction with the participant, the interview process and what the participant said during the interview. The audiotapes need to be transcribed, which is a time-consuming activity if done by the interviewer (although this activity is not without benefits, as we will discuss in the next chapter), and costly if a transcriptionist is hired to type the taped interviews.

Each qualitative interview has its own unique properties and is the antithesis of standardized and replicable. The researcher seeks to generate authentic information by building a relationship of trust with the participant, waiting and negotiating. It is not a process that can be hurried. Participants will construct their own narratives based on the information and experiences they have to date and choose what they do, and do not, want to reveal (Nunkoosing, 2005). It is also worth remembering that accounts of actions and behaviors represent participants' interpretation of what they or others did and will not necessarily correspond with observational data (Britten, 2000). In addition, some participants will be more articulate and able to reflect on events, beliefs and attitudes than others.

In-depth interviewing is a very important qualitative data collection method and, as such, we considered it worth providing a detailed discussion. Many of the issues we have raised are applicable to other data collection methods, such as focus groups.

Focus groups

The focus group method, also known as a focused discussion or group interview, 'is essentially a qualitative data gathering technique that relies upon the systematic questioning of several individuals simultaneously in a formal or informal setting' (Fontana & Frey, 2000, p. 651) and in health care it is characterized by the explicit use of group interaction to generate data. In the past, focus groups were primarily associated with marketing, organizational and community development and the social sciences. However, in recent years focus groups have become an increasingly popular method in health research, although their use 'tended to be confined to hypothesis generation; testing and implementation in the preliminary stages of a project; developing questionnaires; interpreting quantitative results; or designing intervention programs' (Barbour, 2005, p. 742).

Focus groups, like in-depth interviews, can explore the experiences, opinions, attitudes and concerns of participants. Within a focus group, participants can interact with each other in sharing accounts, information and points of view, and generate their own questions and concepts using their own language and vocabulary (Lehoux *et al.*, 2006). Focus groups can facilitate an examination of different perspectives within a common social or cultural network and explore how these are constructed and expressed. They can identify and highlight cultural values or group norms. By observing and analyzing the type of narrative employed, or use of humor and the consensus or dissent that develops within the group, the researcher can identify shared knowledge and common patterns of interaction (Pope & Mays, 2000). From a practical perspective, focus groups enable the researcher to generate a large amount of rich data in a limited period of time and are relatively inexpensive to conduct (Morgan, 1998; Morgan & Scannell, 1998; Barbour & Kitzinger, 1999; Kitzinger, 2005).

There has been a considerable proliferation of rehabilitation literature, including that of occupational therapy and physical therapy (for example Sim & Snell, 1996; Hollis *et al.*, 2002) that discusses the merits and issues of conducting focus group research. There are also many resources addressing the practicalities and skills needed to conduct focus group research and an increasing number of published studies in the rehabilitation literature using a focus group method (for example Boswell *et al.*, 1998; Pain *et al.*, 1998; Toms & Harrison, 2002; Talbot *et al.*, 2004). Similar to the studies described earlier that used an in-depth interview method, this literature mostly discusses the focus group method as a research entity in itself and fails to provide any discussion linking the choice of method to the research purpose and underlying qualitative methodology. As Barbour (2005) suggests, the lack of methodological debate may dilute the capacity of focus group methods to provide valuable insights unless a more critical perspective is adopted to ensure that the choice and design of focus groups is congruent with the dominant qualitative paradigm of the study in question. In an ethnographic study, fieldwork settings provide informal occasions, for example the street corner or a therapy department waiting room, in which informants can be brought together for casual but purposive inquiries. Such focus groups may enable the researcher to solicit explanation or clarification for observed interactions or behavior and can be used for triangulation purposes in conjunction with other data gathering techniques (Fontana & Frey, 2000). A more formal setting and approach to conducting focus groups might be utilized when the research purpose is phenomenological, that is, the intent is to establish the widest range of *intersubjective* meanings and interpretations of a topic.

The skills that are required to conduct a focus group interview are not significantly different from those discussed earlier in relation to in-depth interviewing, but the practicalities of managing group interactions can present some distinctive concerns that group facilitators or moderators may need to address. Much is written about conducting a focus group (for example Sim & Snell, 1996; Pope & Mays, 2000) and the need to subtly control the group dynamics. The importance of the planning and organization stages is evident from the literature, which describes such activities as accessing informants and the involvement of *gatekeepers*, informing the respondents, choosing a suitable location, arranging travel and coordinating informants, deciding how to record the discussion (using a tape recorder or flipchart), and involving an additional person to make notes and document on the flipchart (Morgan, 1998; Barbour & Kitzinger, 1999). In general, facilitating the focus group process means ensuring that 'one person or small coalition of persons' do not dominate the discussion; that informants are encouraged to participate; and that all informants contribute in order to get the fullest coverage of the topic (Fontana & Frey, 2000, p. 652). In our experience, keeping too much control undermines the participants' ability to mediate themselves and total anarchy is unlikely since all those involved in the focus groups have a common interest in sharing what they know or understand about the topic of interest and are likely to avoid unpleasant behavior or confrontation.

Focus groups used in qualitative research tend to be small in size, involving six to ten participants, and can involve strangers, or people who know each other, such as friends or colleagues. These decisions depend on factors such as the research purpose, the amount each individual has to contribute to the topic of interest, how much the researcher wants to hear from each participant and the quality of the group interaction desired (Morgan, 1998; MacDougall & Fudge, 2001). If the group is too small, it can be disrupted more easily by group dynamics, for example the presence of friends, 'experts', or non-participating individuals. Morgan (1998) recommends basing these decisions on the research purpose and the researcher's prior knowledge of the participants and then over-recruiting by 20% to cover for the inevitable no-shows. Focus group interviews usually last one to two hours and some form of question guide is recommended in order to maintain the group's attention on the topic of interest. The purpose of the guide and the role of the moderator are to maintain the flow of the discussion and to channel it, without constraining the discussion (Morgan & Scannell, 1998; Barbour & Kitzinger, 1999; Pope & Mays, 2000).

The definitions of a focus group are relatively vague, for example 'a group discussion exploring a specific set of issues' (Barbour & Kitzinger, 1999), which 'capitalizes on the interaction that occurs within the group setting' (Sim & Snell, 1996). These non-specific definitions and the lack of methodological foundation characteristic of many 'focus group' studies have resulted in confusion and a lack of consistency in the way they are used. In addition, the consensus methods, Delphi technique and nominal group method are occasionally included in descriptions of the focus group method. We prefer to discuss them as separate approaches as they have clearly defined aims, outcomes and processes that differentiate them from focus groups.

Consensus methods

Consensus methods are increasingly being used in occupational therapy and physical therapy (for example Sumsion, 1999; Barclay-Goddard, 2001; Barker & Burns, 2001; Deane *et al.*, 2003) to establish the extent of professional agreement, and in some cases to develop it, when there is a lack of definitive knowledge or evidence about the effectiveness and appropriateness of rehabilitation interventions or other aspects of professional practice, and to develop practice guidelines. Perhaps more than any of the other methods discussed in this chapter, consensus techniques appear to have little or no association with qualitative methodological approaches. Studies utilizing these techniques do so with a focused outcome in mind, for example prioritizing the learning needs of physiotherapy and occupational therapy staff (Barclay-Goddard & Strock, 2001), rather than an exploration of the process of prioritization and decision-making. Consensus techniques could also be used as a method to generate data at a specific stage of a larger participatory action research process. However, we have found no examples of such a use of consensus techniques and it is customary for researchers to use these techniques in a sense as both methodology and method.

There are two main approaches to establishing consensus, the *Delphi technique* (sometimes called Delphi survey approach) and the *nominal group* method. These methods are frequently used in combination (for example MacDonald *et al.*, 2001). Each technique facilitates the qualitative assessment of evidence while deriving quantitative estimates from the evidence (Jones & Hunter, 2000; Bowling & Ebrahim, 2005). The aim of these techniques, as initially conceived, was to canvass expert opinion in order to provide a basis for structured decision-making and forecasting in business and marketing. The Rand Corporation developed the Delphi technique in 1944, and in 1950 made it famous (or infamous) by using it to determine the potential effects and outcomes of an atomic attack on the United States (Helmer, 1967). These consensus techniques 'seek to maximize the benefits from having informed panels consider a problem while minimizing the disadvantages associated with collective decision-making' (Jones & Hunter, 2000, p. 40). As a result, consensus techniques are highly structured and explicit approaches to aggregating participants' responses.

The Delphi technique

The Delphi technique is fundamentally a multi-stage survey process where each stage or round builds on the results of the previous one (Sumsion, 1998). At each stage or round, a questionnaire, developed by the research team, is distributed to participants. Traditionally, round one is used to explore the topic of interest and generate ideas about it, but a more recent approach has entailed providing pre-existing information for the participants to rank and comment on (Sumsion, 1998). At successive rounds, information from the previous questionnaire responses is collated, summarized and included in a repeat version of the questionnaire. This is subsequently redistributed to the participants for further ranking and comment. In successive rounds, the re-rankings are summarized and assessed for the degree of consensus. There appears to be no definitive recommendation about the number of rounds to reach consensus. Traditionally, the Delphi technique consisted of four rounds (Helmer, 1967) but there can be as many as seven rounds

(Sumsion, 1998). In health care research, a maximum of three rounds seems to be common. It is important to define the acceptable degree of consensus established for the study and if this is achieved the final results are distributed to the participants; if not, further rounds are conducted (Jones & Hunter, 2000). There are two types of agreement: first, the extent to which each participant agrees with the stated issue, usually documented on a numerical or categorical scale, and second, the extent to which the participants agree with each other, usually assessed using descriptive statistics (Jones & Hunter, 2000).

The number of participants required for a Delphi technique varies considerably; for example, Barker & Burns (2001) involved an expert panel of 12 physiotherapists, whereas Deane *et al.* (2003) recruited 169 occupational therapists in their study to determine best practice for Parkinson's disease in the UK. There appear to be no guidelines about the optimal number of participants in Delphi technique research, but it is clear that a greater number requires additional resources, in terms of administration and data management. As Sumsion (1998) suggests, 'the process of choosing the participants poses some interesting questions' (p. 154) as traditionally those involved are identified as "experts". For professions like occupational therapy and physical therapy, where a system of formal recognition of practice specialists has not been established, identifying "experts" depends more on their potential contribution to the research topic and their perceived commitment to the profession. Participants can be recruited because of their years of experience working in a particular practice area (Barker & Burns, 2001) or because they are representative of the professional group whose practice is the focus of the research (Sumsion, 1999; Barclay-Goddard, 2001). As well, participants can be recruited because they are members of a professional organization (Deane *et al.*, 2003), have a publication record, are recognized researchers or professional leaders.

There are a number of advantages associated with the Delphi technique. Participants can be recruited from a wide geographical area and do not meet other participants, thus confidentiality can be strictly maintained. Computer technology and the Internet make data management and dissemination of the results of each round to the participant quick, efficient and relatively inexpensive. As with other methods, the credibility of the research findings depends on a rigorous approach to questionnaire construction and data analysis. This technique requires considerable commitment on the part of the participants. As they become more involved with each round their interest and motivation to sustain the process can grow. In contrast, after two or three rounds, participants have been found to become fatigued with the process.

Nominal group method

The nominal group method can be defined as a highly structured focus group brought together to achieve a specific goal. It involves bringing together a number (usually 9–12) of experts in the area of interest. This focus is typically well-defined, for example to develop consensus on the appropriateness of physical therapy interventions in cardiorespiratory practice or determine curricular priorities to support the change from baccalaureate to graduate professional degrees. The nominal group process is facilitated either by an individual who is an expert on the topic or a credible non-expert (Jones & Hunter, 2000) and a second person may be involved to act as recorder and observer of the group process. The technique consists of at least two rounds in which the group members define their opinions, discuss, rate and then re-rate a series of ideas or concepts. The process begins by the group individually recording their opinions on the topic and contributing one idea to the facilitator. Ideas are recorded on a flipchart, post-it notes or a computer and then these ideas are grouped, clarified and evaluated by the participants. After a thorough discussion, each group member privately ranks each idea. These rankings are tabulated and presented by the facilitator for further discussion, followed by further re-rankings and so on, until group consensus has been reached. The nominal technique is clearly focused on achieving a specified outcome. The facilitator takes a more directive role and data analysis is immediate and part of the process. The same issues of participant recruitment arise in the nominal group method as discussed in relation to the Delphi technique.

We have briefly described consensus techniques in this section and for those interested in conducting this type of research we recommend a number of resources (Walker & Selfe, 1996; Murphy, 1998; Sumsion, 1998; Jones & Hunter, 2000) in which these techniques are discussed in more detail. There is some debate about the validity and applicability of these techniques, and Jones & Hunter (2000) warn of the 'danger that each [technique] has evolved a well-developed structure and sequence of activities, and can often be used to generate quantitative estimates of agreement, [that] may lead the [uncritical] observer to place greater reliance on the results than might be warranted' (p. 48).

Participant observation

Participant observation involves the researcher in a complex process of observing, participating, interrogating, listening, communicating, negotiating, recording and interacting (Mason, 2002), and requires researchers to enter a setting or situation to do fieldwork for a prolonged period of time. It is a more challenging process than conducting in-depth interviews because social or cultural settings, situations and interactions can be 'notoriously messy' and complicated, with lots of things happening at once (Mason 2002, p. 87). It requires greater personal investment and time than other methods of data collection. Participant observation can be used as a supplementary or supportive method of data gathering, although it is frequently the primary method in ethnographic studies where the main aim is descriptive (Robson, 2002).

The first task of the researcher is to locate a context or setting (or field) from which data relevant to the research question or aim can be generated. Unless the researcher is an insider, access to a setting or group is usually negotiated with the assistance of a gatekeeper. This person is usually in a position to support and promote the research and to negotiate with members of the group on the researcher's behalf (see Chapter 4 for more discussion of this role). Having gained access to the research setting the researcher needs to spend some time initially 'striking up sufficient rapport and empathy with the group to enable the study to be conducted' (Pope & Mays, 2000, p. 34). At this stage it is also important to decide on what Angrosino (2005) calls the researcher's *situational identity* or what Coffey (1999) refers to as the *ethnographic self*. In health care research it is rarely, if ever, acceptable for researchers to conduct research in a covert manner by concealing their real purpose for interacting within the group. A deliberate and planned intention to deceive participants is regarded as indefensible and would not gain institutional ethics approval (Robson, 2002).

A number of alternative observational roles have been identified (Robson, 2002; Wallace, 2005). The *detached observer* does not interact with the group even though their status as a researcher has been established. Superficially, the concept of the neutral observer is appealing, but in reality it is generally not desirable or feasible. The *marginal participant* role is achieved by keeping a low profile. Robson (2002) describes the researcher in this role as a largely passive, though familiar and accepted, presence rather like a passenger on a train observing the other passengers. The presence of 'an observer may stimulate modifications in behavior and action – the so-called Hawthorne effect – although this is seen to reduce over time' (Pope & Mays, 2000, p. 34). Angrosino (2005) suggests that since the purpose of research utilizing participant observation is usually to gain an in-depth understanding of social interaction, it makes no sense for the researcher to be a passive observer. Angrosino (2005) recommends that the researcher seek a *situational identity* based on membership or participation. In this role the researcher fully informs the group of the observer role being taken, but in addition establishes close relationships with members of the group by assuming a recognized role, for example as a volunteer or someone who can repair wheelchairs. This role can build trust and facilitate the researcher selectively asking members to explain various aspects of what is going on. These 'on the wing' discussions or informal interviews can effectively support systematic observation, although over time they may lead to a blurring of the dual roles adopted by the researcher (Robson, 2002, p. 320).

Whatever role researchers adopt, their central task is to turn their observations into data. It can be daunting to know how to organize and select from the bulk of material, information and impressions that can potentially be generated (Mason, 2002). *Field notes* are the primary strategy for recording observations and these may be supplemented, as appropriate, by video recording, audiotaping or photographs. Emerson *et al.* (2001) describe field notes as:

Writings produced in close proximity to 'the field'. Proximity means that field-notes are written more or less *contemporaneously* with the events, experiences and interactions they describe and recount. . . . Field notes are a form of *representation*, that is, a way of reducing just-observed events, persons and places to written accounts (p. 353).

How field notes are written and organized therefore depends on what the researcher is interested in and wants the field notes to represent. Each researcher makes individual decisions about how their field notes are to be formatted and managed. However, these decisions determine how data are to be retrieved, located and conceptualized later in the research process, and whether the researcher can engage in literal, interpretive and reflexive analysis at a later stage (Mason, 2002). Spradley (1980) provides a framework that is often cited as being useful in organizing contextual descriptive data. The framework includes the dimensions of space (physical/places), actors (people), activities (of people), objects (physical things used by people), acts (specific things people do), events (particular occasions involving people), time (sequencing of events), goals (things people are trying to accomplish) and feelings (emotions expressed by people).

Sometimes, note-taking will interfere with the active involvement of the observer or be too intrusive and will need to be developed after the experience. For example, Suto (2000) attended a craft activity with the participants in her ethnographic study exploring temporal perspectives in the roles and occupations of people with chronic schizophrenia. During the activity, she took the opportunity to solicit clarification from the participants and immediately after the event ended she wrote detailed field notes about her observations. Some observers in such situations use memory aids to assist their recall later or jot down key words or phrases as unobtrusively as possible. Others focus on documenting descriptions of critical incidents, that is, discrete events or specific contexts (Pope & Mays, 2000).

In observational methods of data gathering, in particular, the data collection and analytic processes are intertwined. The researcher not only constructs a detailed portrait or narrative account of what is being observed but also develops a conceptual or theoretical framework, grounded in the observational material, which helps the researcher understand and explain to others what is going on. This conceptual framework, in turn, enables the researcher to focus their observations on a specific dimension or themes that cross several dimensions (Robson, 2002). At no time is the concept of researcher as research instrument or tool more apparent than in participant observation, and some of the most challenging debates about qualitative methods have occurred in relation to ethnography and observation and the ethical issues they raise (Mason, 2002).

'Unobtrusive' methods

This section has focused primarily on people (individuals or groups) as the source of data. In health care research, unobtrusive methods of data collection are defined as those that do not actively require the involvement of research participants. 'Unobtrusive' methods can involve accessing information from a variety of sources (Kellehear, 1993), such as:

- *Cultural material*, including physical objects (for example rehabilitation equipment or patient information pamphlets), physical traces (for example discarded paper or signs of wear and tear on equipment) and settings (for example the organization of a rehabilitation ward or unit).

- *The written record*, which could include documents obtained from libraries, individuals, government or organization records, books (health care records, autobiographies or non-fiction accounts) and personal documents, such as diaries and letters. In health care, it is imperative to ensure that the person is fully informed and to obtain that person's permission to access and review personal documents and health care records.
- *The audiovisual record*, including information obtained from films, television programs, videos, images, music and photographs (for example conducting an exploration of how disabled people are portrayed in films and television programs).
- *Simple observation* can be carried out by systematically watching and recording people's behaviors, the way they dress, generally express themselves and interact with others in a particular public location or context (for example an outpatient waiting room or rehabilitation center cafeteria). The important characteristics of simple observation are that the location is public, and that the participants are not engaged or involved in the study in any way and do not interact directly with the researcher.
- *The use of hardware*, by which Kellehear (1993) refers to computers and software packages, could include conducting a literature search and critically appraising relevant research literature.

Unobtrusive methods of data collection are primarily used to supplement other interactive data collection methods in triangulating data sources, for example in ethnographic studies. They are also useful when it is not feasible to collect data through interactive methods because of the sensitive nature of the topic or simply because those who could provide the information are no longer available for the researcher to engage with (Rice & Ezzy, 1999).

Regardless of the choice of data collection method (or methods), or the experience of the researcher, an initial *pilot study* can provide invaluable information by which data gathering can be refined. In general, a pilot study involves conducting a small version of the research process, such as data collection and analysis, and then soliciting feedback from volunteer participants. A *pilot test* is usually focused more on practicing the data collection strategy, for example trying out interview skills, testing some focus group questions, writing and organizing the field notes from a trial observation session.

In this chapter, we have discussed qualitative sampling strategies and a number of data collection methods used in health care research. In qualitative research, the researcher is a tool or instrument; in other words, the researcher is an integral component of the research, and this is clearly reflected in the methods we have discussed, particularly in-depth interviews and participant observation. This role brings with it the responsibility of fully locating ourselves in the research (*positionality*) and engaging in disciplined self-reflection (*reflexivity*). *Positionality* refers to making a full explanation of our experience and knowledge of the research topic, our interest in the topic and our relationship with the participants. *Reflexivity* requires us to evaluate our subjective responses continually throughout the research process and our methodological decision-making. The concepts of positionality and reflexivity are discussed in more detail in Chapter 7. In making decisions about how to recruit and involve participants in research and in choosing a data collection method or methods we are faced with the need to address the important ethical issues of ensuring confidentiality and informed consent, discussed in Chapter 3. In the next chapter, we will discuss the nature and different forms of qualitative data and the practical issues of effectively managing and organizing data.

References

Angrosino, M.V. (2005) Recontextualizing observation: ethnography, pedagogy, and the prospects for a progressive political agenda. In: N.K. Denzin & Y.S. Lincoln (eds), *The Sage Handbook of Qualitative Research* (3rd edn, pp. 729–745). Thousand Oaks, Calif., Sage.

Barbour, R. (2005) Making sense of focus groups. *Medical Education*, 39, 742–750.

Barbour, R. & Kitzinger, J. (eds) (1999) *Developing Focus Group Research*. London, Sage.

Barclay-Goddard, R. & Strock, A. (2001) A collaborative approach to learning needs assessment using the Delphi technique. *Physiotherapy Canada*, Summer, 190–194.

Barker, K. & Burns, M. (2001) Using consensus techniques to produce clinical guidelines for patients treated with the Ilizarov Fixator. *Physiotherapy*, 87 (6), 289–300.

Blank, A. (2004) Clients' experiences of partnership with occupational therapists in community mental health. *British Journal of Occupational Therapy*, 67 (3), 118–124.

Boswell, B.B., Dawson, M. & Heininger, E. (1998) Quality of life as defined by adults with spinal cord injuries. *Journal of Rehabilitation*, January/February/March, 27–32.

Bourke-Taylor, H. & Hudson, D. (2005) Cultural differences: the experience of establishing an occupational therapy service in a developing community. *Australian Occupational Therapy Journal*, 52, 188–198.

Bowling, A. & Ebrahim, S. (eds) (2005) *Handbook of Health Research Methods*. Buckingham, Open University Press.

Britten, N. (2000) Qualitative interviews in health care research. In: C. Pope & N. Mays (eds), *Qualitative Research in Health Care* (2nd edn, pp. 11–29). London, BMJ Books.

Carpenter, C. (1994) The experience of spinal cord injury: the individual's perspective – implications for rehabilitation practice. *Physical Therapy*, 74 (7), 614–629.

Carpenter, C. (2004) Dilemmas of practice as experienced by physical therapists in rehabilitation settings. *Physiotherapy Canada*, 57 (1), 63–74.

Charmaz, K. (2000) Grounded theory: objectivist and constructivist methods. In: N.K. Denzin & Y.S. Lincoln (eds), *Handbook of Qualitative Research* (2nd edn, pp. 509–535). Thousand Oaks, Calif., Sage.

Coffey, A. (1999) *The Ethnographic Self: Fieldwork and the Representation of Identity*. London, Sage.

Deane, K.H.O., Ellis-Hill, C., Dekker, K., Davies, P. & Clarke, C.E. (2003) A Delphi survey of best practice occupational therapy for Parkinson's disease in the United Kingdom. *British Journal of Occupational Therapy*, 66 (6), 247–254.

Emerson, R.M., Fretz, R.I. & Shaw, L.L. (2001) Participant observation and field notes. In: P. Atkinson, A. Coffey, S. Delamount, J. Lofland & L. Lofland (eds), *Handbook of Ethnography* (pp. 453–467). Thousand Oaks, Calif., Sage.

Fontana, A. & Frey, J.H. (2000) The interview: from structured questions to negotiated text. In: N.K. Denzin & Y.S. Lincoln (eds), *Handbook of Qualitative Research* (2nd edn, pp. 645–672). Thousand Oaks, Calif., Sage.

Ford, S., Schofield, T. & Hope, T. (2002) What are the ingredients for a successful evidence-based patient choice consultation? A qualitative study. *Social Science & Medicine*, 56, 589–602.

Glaser, B.G. & Strauss, A.L. (1967) *The Discovery of Grounded Theory: Strategies for Qualitative Research*. Chicago, Aldine.

Helmer, O. (1967) *Convergence of Expert Consensus Through Feedback*. Los Angeles, Rand Corporation.

Hollis, V., Openshaw, S. & Goble, R. (2002) Conducting focus groups: purpose and practicalities. *British Journal of Occupational Therapy*, 65 (1), 65–71.

Jones, J. & Hunter, D. (2000) Using the Delphi and nominal group technique in health services research. In: C. Pope & N. Mays (eds), *Qualitative Research in Health Care* (2nd edn, pp. 40–49). London, BMJ Books.

Kellehear, A. (1993) *The Unobtrusive Researcher: a Guide to Methods*. Sydney, Allen & Unwin.

Kitzinger, J. (2005) Focus group research: using group dynamics to explore perceptions, experiences and understandings. In: I. Holloway (ed.), *Qualitative Research in Health Care* (pp. 56–70). Oxford, Blackwell.

Lehoux, P., Poland, B. & Daudelin, G. (2006) Focus group research and 'the patient's view'. *Social Science & Medicine*, 63, 2091–2104.

Lund, M.L. & Nygaard, L. (2004) Occupational life in the home environment: the experiences of people with disabilities. *Canadian Journal of Occupational Therapy*, 71 (4), 243–251.

MacDonald, C.A., Houghton, P., Cox, P.D. & Bartlett, D. (2001) Consensus on physical therapy professional behaviors. *Physiotherapy Canada*, Summer, 212–222.

MacDougall, C.A. & Fudge, E. (2001) Planning and recruiting the sample for focus groups and in-depth interviews. *Qualitative Health Research*, 11 (1), 117–126.

MacLean, N., Pound, P., Wolfe, C. & Rudd, C. (2000) Qualitative analysis of stroke patients' motivation for rehabilitation. *British Medical Journal*, 321 (28 October), 1051–1054.

Marquis, R. & Jackson, R. (2000) Quality of life and quality of service relationships: experiences of people with disabilities. *Disability & Society*, 15 (3), 411–425.

Mason, J. (2002) *Qualitative Researching* (2nd edn). London, Sage.

Miles, M. & Hubermann, A. (1994) *Qualitative Data Analysis: an Expanded Sourcebook* (2nd edn). Newbury Park, Calif., Sage.

Miller W.L. & Crabtree B.F. (2005) Clinical research. In: N.K. Denzin & Y.S. Lincoln (eds), *The Sage Handbook of Qualitative Research* (pp. 605–639). Thousand Oaks, Calif., Sage.

Morgan, D.L. (1998) *The Focus Group Guidebook*. Thousand Oaks, Calif., Sage.

Morgan, D.L. & Scannell, A.U. (1998) *Planning Focus Groups*. Thousand Oaks, Calif., Sage.

Morse, J.M. (1998). What's wrong with random selection? *Qualitative Health Research*, 8 (6), 733–735.

Morse, J.M. (2000) Editorial: determining sample size. *Qualitative Health Research*, 10 (1), 3–5.

Morse, J.M. & Field, P.A. (1995) *Qualitative Research Methods for Health Professionals.* Thousand Oaks, Calif., Sage.

Murphy, M.K., Black, N.A., Lamping, D.L. *et al.* (1998) Consensus development methods and their use in clinical guideline development. *Health Technology Assessment*, 2 (3), 1–87.

Nunkoosing, K. (2005) The problems with interviews. *Qualitative Health Research*, 15 (5), 698–706.

Pain, K., Dunn, M., Anderson, G., Darrah, J. & Kratochvil, M. (1998) Quality of life: what does it mean in rehabilitation? *Journal of Rehabilitation*, April/May/June, 5–11.

Patton, M.Q. (2002) *Qualitative Research & Evaluation Methods* (3rd edn). Thousand Oaks, Calif., Sage.

Pope, C. & Mays, N. (eds) (2000) *Qualitative Research in Health Care* (2nd edn). London, BMJ Books.

Rice, P.L. & Ezzy, D. (1999) *Qualitative Research Methods.* Oxford, Oxford University Press.

Ritchie, J. (2001) Case series research: a case for qualitative method in assembling evidence. *Physiotherapy Theory and Practice*, 17, 127–135.

Robson, C. (2002) *Real World Research* (2nd edn). Oxford, Blackwell.

Rubin, H.J. & Rubin I.S. (2005) *Qualitative Interviewing: the Art of Hearing Data* (2nd edn). Thousand Oaks, Calif., Sage.

Sandelowski, M. (2002) Keynote address: re-embodying qualitative enquiry. *Qualitative Health Research*, 12 (1), 104–115.

Schacter, C., Stalker, C. & Teram, E. (1999) Toward sensitive practice: issues for physical therapists working with survivors of childhood abuse. *Physical Therapy*, 79 (3), 248–261.

Scheer, J., Kroll, T., Neri, M.T. & Beatty, P. (2003) Access barriers for persons with disabilities: the consumer's perspective. *Journal of Disability Policy Studies*, 13 (4), 221–230.

Sim, J. & Snell, J. (1996) Focus groups in physiotherapy evaluation and research. *Physiotherapy*, 82 (3), 189–198.

Spradley, J.P. (1980) *Participant Observation.* New York, Holt, Rinehart & Winston.

Stake, R.E. (2000) Case studies. In: N.K. Denzin & Y.S. Lincoln (eds), *Handbook of Qualitative Research* (2nd edn, pp. 435–454). Thousand Oaks, Calif., Sage.

Strauss, A. & Corbin, J. (1990) *Basics of Qualitative Research: Grounded Theory Procedures and Techniques.* Newbury Park, Calif., Sage.

Stringer, E. & Genat, W.J. (2004) *Action Research in Health.* Peer Saddle River, NJ, Pearson/Merrill Prentice Hall.

Sumsion, T. (1998) The Delphi technique: an adaptive research tool. *British Journal of Occupational Therapy*, 61 (4), 153–156.

Sumsion, T. (1999) A study to determine a British occupational therapy definition of client-centered practice. *British Journal of Occupational Therapy*, 62 (2), 52–58.

Suto, M. (2000) Issues related to data collection. In: K.W. Hammell, C. Carpenter & I. Dyck (eds), *Using Qualitative Research: a Practical Introduction for Occupational and Physical Therapists* (pp. 35–46). Edinburgh, Churchill Livingstone.

Talbot, K.R., Viscogliosi, C., Desrosiers, J., Vincent, C., Rousseau, J. & Robichaud, L. (2004) Identification of rehabilitation needs after a stroke: an exploratory study. *Health and Quality of Life Outcomes*, 2, 53–62.

Taylor, M.C. (2005) Interviewing. In: I. Holloway (ed.), *Qualitative Research in Health Care* (pp. 39–55). Oxford, Blackwell.

Teddlie, C. & Yu, F. (2007) Mixed method sampling: a typology with examples. *Journal of Mixed Methods Research*, *1* (1), 77–100.

Toms, J. & Harrison, K. (2002) Living with chronic lung disease and the effect of rehabilitation: patients' perspectives. *Physiotherapy*, *88* (10), 605–619.

Walker, A.M. & Selfe, J. (1996) The Delphi method: a useful tool for the allied health researcher. *British Journal of Therapy and Rehabilitation*, *3* (12), 677–681.

Wallace, S. (2005) Observing method: recognizing the significance of belief, discipline, position and documentation in observational studies. In: I. Holloway (ed.), *Qualitative Research in Health Care* (pp. 71–89). Oxford, Blackwell.

Yin, R. (2003) *Case Study Research: Design and Methods* (3rd edn). Thousand Oaks, Calif., Sage.

Chapter 6
MANAGING QUALITATIVE DATA

Introduction

The intent of this chapter is to demonstrate how to organize, retrieve and present data in forms that are consistent with the aims of qualitative research. We build on the discussion of data collection methods, such as interviews and participant observation provided in the previous chapter, to outline processes that prepare the data for analysis. Interviews are transcribed into data in text-based form and data such as photographs or video recordings may be used in their original form. *Transcription* is a unique feature of qualitative research and there are choices to make about the style of transcription as well as the role that the *transcriptionist* plays. Researchers should recognize that all media eventually become obsolete and choose the best archival format for their data. In different stages of the research process, each decision taken should be examined for its compatibility with the purposes of qualitative research: discovery, description and exploration of human life and social relations (Denzin & Lincoln, 2005). Choices about how to handle data reflect strategies the researcher uses to support the individual or group perspective central to qualitative research and prepare for the analytic and interpretive phases of inquiry. The management of copious data is challenging and computer-assisted analysis of qualitative data systems (CAQDAS) offers efficiencies for storage, coding and organization. Alternative strategies for managing the data are presented, which may fit a research project best when there is no access to CAQDAS or there is a preference for using a word processing program.

Qualitative data are generated in a particular context that encompasses the participant and the researcher, their relationship, the immediate milieu, and the influence of social, cultural and physical environments. An important aspect of transferring data into suitable forms for analysis is to provide contextual enrichment through various means: writing up research protocols, creating field notes and maintaining a detailed research journal or field diary (Flick, 2006). What constitutes data is a decision that researchers make each time they select which observations are worthy of writing up as field notes, what content is relevant to transcribe from audiotaped interviews, and when to activate recording equipment such as video cameras. The sensitizing concepts that the researcher is working with and the research question help direct the researcher's gaze towards some potential data and away from others; we view these as interpretive choices.

Morse & Richards (2002) propose ways in which careful attention to good data management can redirect the inquiry. First, this may occur when data 'demand to be treated by a particular method' (p. 106), for example if field notes from participant observations show that the participants are engaging the researcher in long, descriptive conversations that the researcher cannot document accurately. This suggests the need for individual audiotaped interviews. Second, good data management helps the researcher identify what remains to be known or understood. Writing questions at the end of field notes may direct the researcher to seek out documents, ask key informants questions, or observe particular activities. Third, attention to the data that the researcher is creating may reveal that some data collection methods are unworkable or unlikely to produce credible findings. Consider, for example, a study in which the researcher plans to interview together a client who is in the early stages of dementia and her or his family caregiver. If the family caregiver speaks frequently for the person with dementia and does not allow that person the opportunity to contribute, then this data creation method would need to be reassessed.

Different types of qualitative data

Audiotaping

Given the popularity of interviewing in qualitative research, we will first discuss how audiotaping creates a bridge between the interactive but transitory social interaction that defines an interview and the two-dimensional transcripts that are formed from it. Audiotaping is the primary means of recording qualitative interviews that occur in person and over the telephone and it may also be used to capture focus group discussions. The value of having good quality recording equipment, checking the sound level of the recorded voices and bringing extra batteries or an extension cord is immeasurable. Tips about the mechanics of audiotaping were presented in Chapter 3 and becoming skilled with the technology allows the researcher to attend more closely to the content and process of the interview. Although recording devices can seem intrusive initially, a skilled interviewer can diminish the initial discomfort or intimidation that some participants may feel through rapport building and the manner in which the interview unfolds. Fostering a dialogue with the participant, rather than simply asking questions and writing down the answers, contributes to an exploration of issues and the co-construction of knowledge that is the aim of many research projects. The advantages of audiotaping include the creation of an accurate record of what was said, and a sense of the relationship between the participant and the researcher. It also decreases the likelihood of prematurely interpreting or summarizing the data, which would be inappropriate at this stage.

Audiotapes and digital recordings are converted into text through transcription that typically involves listening to and word processing the entire interview. There are also software programs that allow the transcriptionist to listen to the interview and read it into a microphone attached to the computer, which then produces text. Morse & Richards (2002) contend that the transcription of audiotapes is not just mechanical but interpretive and therefore the person who transcribes requires training and some understanding of the research. When making decisions

Table 6.1 Transcription questions.

- Who should transcribe the interview?
- What should the transcript look like?
- When should the interview be transcribed?
- Where will the transcript be stored?
- Why are verbatim transcripts valuable?

---

about transcribing interviews, a researcher may wish to consider the questions in Table 6.1.

Who should transcribe the interview?

For unfunded research, the researcher is the most likely person to transcribe the audiotaped interviews into text. This choice, although an intensive activity, has a number of advantages. Doing the transcription oneself offers the best chance that the content, punctuation and tone of the interview are reflected in the transcript. In studies with small numbers of participant interviews, we have done our own transcription and, like Laliberte-Rudman & Moll (2001), used the transcription process to identify changes that should be made to the interview and to formulate early analytic ideas through memos (Suto, 2000; Carpenter, 2004). Transcription can also be viewed as an interpretive act. It enables the researcher to become thoroughly familiar with the data and 'facilitates the close attention and the interpretive thinking that is needed to make sense of the data' (Lapadat & Lindsay cited by Bird, 2005, p. 230). In this way, the act of transcribing the data becomes integral to the analytic process. Even if the researcher does not transcribe the data, the assumption is that they will have direct supervision of the transcription process and provide guidance to the person who does assume that role (Bird, 2005).

A paid transcriptionist is costly, but the quality and speed of the transcription and researcher's time saved may influence this decision. Estimates of transcription time range from four to eight hours for every one-hour of audiotaped interview (Green & Thorogood, 2004). This range depends on typing speed, transcription style, quality of the recording, accented speech and other factors. The decision about who should transcribe is premised upon the methodology chosen, the anticipated number of interviews and the content of the interviews. In studying health determinants, Meadows *et al.* (2003) found that disturbing stories of 'violence, death, discrimination and economics are potentially raised' (p. 14), noting that these stories are not exclusive to Aboriginal populations. The likelihood of content that may be disturbing to the transcriptionist has implications for training and the incorporation of periodic debriefing. Later in this chapter, we address the benefits and drawbacks of doing one's own transcription versus hiring a professional.

What should the transcript look like?

The look of the transcript is influenced by the methodological theory, the type of coding and strategy for analysis. Grounded theory analysis typically begins with

Table 6.2 Sample interview transcript.

Participant #02	Interview 1/2	4 January 2007	L. Smythe

LS: I'm interested in your experience using the Handi-Dart transportation to go where you need to. Can you tell me what it was like the last time the service gave you a lift?

021:    Well I had to, you know, book about a year in advance. No, just kidding, but there's no chance of any spontaneous trips with Handi-Dart. [cough] I don't mean to be ungrateful and, but you see I phoned four days ahead to get to my daughter in Surrey – is this what you want to know or am I getting too picky with details?

LS: No it's grand, for this project the more details the better, so carry on. Would you like some water?

021:    I'm fine, no. Where was, oh yeah the planning. They could only pick me up at uhm 9.30 'cause of scheduling other people and so I bundled up and hauled myself outside at oh, 9.20 and you wouldn't believe what time they arrived. 10.25! I was just about ready to [word? spit] in a bucket, I was so mad. Sometimes I think they think we don't have nothing better to do because we're not working and maybe they don't realize I paid taxes for years and deserve help now that I'm in this contraption [taps wheelchair].

LS: Oh my. What did you do while you were waiting?

021:    Well, I was freezing, so by about 10 or maybe a few minutes after, I went back inside, no mean feat with the snow and this chair, and rang the, whatcha the, the dispatch office.

LS: What happened then? What did they say?

C:/Smythe/Research/SCI/Interviews.doc

line-by-line coding and each line of text is numbered for ease of identification and retrieval (Pope, *et al.*, 2006). Researchers using thematic analysis, which is associated with phenomenology and ethnography, may choose to have the text displayed in paragraph format, as codes may be assigned to larger chunks of data (Bogdan & Biklen, 2003). Whatever display the researcher selects, it is helpful to create a face sheet for documenting standard information and to follow a consistent format for the layout of the text (Flick, 2006). A consistent format includes indicators of who is speaking; one and a half or double line spaced text, pagination, headers or footers; an ample margin on one side of the page for coding; and a notation system for unclear or missed words, laughter, affirmative utterances (um-hum), length of silences and interruptions. Table 6.2 shows an example of an interview transcript segment. Transcripts are displayed in various ways and choices should be informed by how the transcript will serve the data analysis.

When should the interview be transcribed?

It is advisable to conduct a pilot test of the interview for the purpose of getting feedback on the researcher's interviewing technique, the time allotted for interviews and the utility of the questions and in this situation transcription should occur as soon as possible after the interview. Again, the methodology a researcher uses has some influence on when interviews should be transcribed. If the researcher is using grounded theory, where the data generation and analysis is an iterative and simultaneous process, transcription should be done as soon as possible because it informs the developing concepts. If the data generation methods include more than interviews, as with ethnographic research using participant observation, the timing of transcription may be delayed as field notes are written and guide further data generation.

Where will the transcript be stored?

Transcripts are typically stored in password-protected files and printed for data analysis purposes. Printed documents are stored in locked filing cabinets or in equally secure locations that are detailed on the informed consent document. Regardless of measures to ensure anonymity, careless handling of transcripts could allow someone to identify the research participant through clues in the transcript, such as place of employment, people mentioned, the participant names and specific events that have occurred in the participant's neighbourhood. As with client health records, interview transcripts must be treated confidentially to ensure privacy.

Why are verbatim transcripts valuable?

Verbatim transcripts reproduce word for word the talk and verbalizations of all parties within interview situations. Transcription of the dialogue between the participant (or focus group members) and the researcher allows researchers to analyze the meaning-making process and the role they play in it (Hesse-Biber & Leavy, 2006). Identifying how the researcher is shaping the data generation prompts modifications in the interview style and provides data for the reflexive process. The exact way that participants speak and engage in dialogue may be more or less relevant to the research question. Phrases such as 'like' or 'you know?' may be innocuous fillers of no analytic consequence or they may signal hesitation, an uncertainty or implicit agreement with the interviewer. For practical reasons, some researchers advocate transcribing only what is relevant to the research topic (Flick, 2006); others suggest transcribing the first few interviews verbatim and then omitting superfluous conversations and utterances in subsequent transcriptions (Bogdan & Biklen, 2003). We value verbatim transcription whenever possible and recognize that 'what is relevant' is not always apparent early in a project.

Videotaping

Videotaping is common in Western societies and familiar to people through its use in recording weddings, family gatherings and other events (Bogdan & Biklen, 2003). Typically used in conjunction with other data generation methods, videotaping can capture social processes such as therapy sessions, children's play and other kinds of interactions. The use of video cameras is criticized as being intrusive and changing what people say and do; this criticism is also leveled at participant observation. Bogdan & Biklen (2003) suggest that the effects of video-taping (or still photography) can be minimized by the frequency of the technology in the setting; people often habituate to it over time. People who are busy doing activities are less likely to attend to the camera, although there may be some early sessions where the distraction factor is obvious. Obtaining consent from all participants that are subject to being videotaped can be challenging. Murphy & Dingwall (2003) caution that videotaping can create a huge amount of data, particularly if the researcher is not clear about what is important to record. When videotaping, there may be a false sense that one has documented the reality of the setting and social interactions when in fact each researcher selects what is worthy of recording, which is seldom the 'whole picture' (Flick, 2006).

Parry (2006) used videotaping in her study of how physiotherapists and stroke patients communicate with each other about the activities of therapy during treatment sessions. Although data generation was relatively quick, Parry spent many weeks reviewing the interactions and writing descriptive summaries of each episode. She chose to transcribe the conversations and the movements of particular episodes into written text. There are protocols for transcribing videotapes for conversation analysis and Parry used a free computer program called *Transana* to assist with all aspects of data preparation. Videotaping holds considerable promise for research in rehabilitation settings, where clients and therapists may already be accustomed to observation by students or family members. Mattingly & Fleming's (1994) study of clinical reasoning in occupational therapy provides an excellent example of how videotape may be used, in conjunction with interviews, to make explicit previously discussed cognitive and interactive processes.

Field notes

The purpose of field notes is to create 'a description of people, objects, places, events, activities, and conversations' (Bogdan & Biklen, 2003, p. 110). In ethnographic research, field notes are the product of participant observation and a primary method for generating data. The use of field notes has permeated other methodological approaches, such as grounded theory, where understanding social processes is the focus. Researchers may also write field notes after interviews to describe the setting and the process of the interview, as well as to record their impressions. Writing field notes takes time, discipline and a good memory; the latter improves with practice. Most researchers emphasize the importance of writing field notes within hours of the observation and avoiding any discussion about the observations, as that may dilute one's impressions or prompt writing that is too interpretative at this stage (Lofland *et al.*, 2006). Good field notes are concrete, behavioral, descriptive and chronological.

Field notes often begin as jottings in the setting when the researcher writes key words, phrasings or bits of conversation that will later prompt recall of what occurred. Field notes taken during participant observation are called 'a condensed account' (Spradley, 1980, p. 69) as they reflect a running chronology of what happened, who interacted with whom and at what time. Hammersley & Atkinson (1995) note that participant observers, in their attempts to write unobtrusively, make frequent use of the bathroom on site to obtain privacy for quick jottings. Other spaces where one may write uninterrupted work equally well. Accurate note-taking is important and may include detailed maps of the setting and other graphic representations that show where social processes occur and who is involved. For example, a rehabilitation professional observing participants in a clinic would describe the clinic layout, indicate the location of all items, identify and describe who was in the clinic, and what they were doing and saying. The researcher would avoid generalities, such as 'it was a typically large, outpatient clinic where physiotherapy and occupational therapy services were offered'. Field notes written early in a project describe everything about the setting because what is most important is not yet clear. Subsequent field notes document changes in the setting and begin to focus on what the researcher decides is of interest, a decision that occurs through sensitizing concepts and reviews of previous field notes.

In creating an accurate and useful set of field notes consider Spradley's (1980) position that 'the moment you begin writing down what you see and hear, you automatically encode things in language . . . the language used in field notes has numerous long-term consequences for your research' (pp. 64–65). Thus, the language that you use to write should reflect the different types of communication that you hear. In some settings, for example, there is variation between the jargon and speech patterns used by service providers and service recipients. It is important to retain these variations when documenting verbatim or paraphrased material as they may reflect cultural meanings (even if the 'culture' is a hospital or clinic). Suto (2000), in her board and care home research, was aware of four languages (all English) that shaped how she wrote field notes. First, there was her language that was influenced by advanced education and professional socialization. Second, there was the language of social science, full of abstractions and new perspectives, which Suto was learning as she conducted the research. Third, there was the language of the participants who had severe chronic mental illnesses that was distinguished by particular jargon. Fourth, there was the language of the staff that does not fit any of the other ways of talking. When writing the 'expanded account' of field notes Spradley (1980) advises researchers to 'expand, fill out, enlarge, and give as much specific detail as possible' (p. 68) in order to keep the data grounded in the setting. Novice researchers might choose to avoid repeating descriptions of recurrent events, but upon analysis, such repetition sometimes illuminates patterns of behavior or cultural meanings.

Full field notes should be written using a consistent format that facilitates ease of reading, retrieval, coding and analytic choices (see Table 6.3 for an example). Field notes for each observation (or post-interview) have a heading on the first page that includes date and location of the observation, duration, field notes number in a series and a summary of the session (Bogdan & Biklen, 2003). We recommend that researchers write in paragraphs, paginate, insert a header or footer and allow a large margin for coding. If the analysis requires line-by-line coding then we suggest using the line number formatting standard to most word

Table 6.3 Field notes example.

<table>
<tr><td colspan="2" align="center">Field notes (expanded account)</td><td colspan="2"></td></tr>
<tr><td>Date:</td><td>12 August 1993</td><td>OC:</td><td>Observer's comments</td></tr>
<tr><td>Location:</td><td>Crestview board and care</td><td>PC:</td><td>Participant's comments</td></tr>
<tr><td>Duration:</td><td>11.00 am–2.15pm</td><td colspan="2">Verbatim quote: "double quote"</td></tr>
<tr><td>Week:</td><td>#1/10</td><td colspan="2">Paraphrased talk: 'single quote'</td></tr>
<tr><td>Field notes:</td><td>#2/30</td><td colspan="2"></td></tr>
</table>

Summary of observations
Talked to Tony (administrator) for the first 15 minutes re: consents, chart access, then wandered the first floor saying hello to people I'd met last time. Watched TV for $1/2$ hour, had lunch with group, got three more consents (Arlan, Phil, John). Attended the arts and crafts group with six people; owner's cousin led group (45 minutes).

Narrative	Coding

11:00 Another warm summer morning. I'm grateful that we're not having the deadly 100F+ weather like last month. I feel more comfortable here this week; as I was feeding money in the meter I saw Mr Y and he greeted me by name. Walked in the lobby past the plastic flowers and into the ever-present smoke haze. The cooks (LS, DT) and the cleaning man (JT) said hello to me (buenos dias – JT) when I walked in to put my lunch in the fridge.

Approached TK (administrator) who was drinking a can of Pepsi and asked if we could talk sometime in next two hours, "Let's do it now". (PC) He's wearing Bermuda shorts, birkinstocks and a yellow T-shirt. Went into his office and presented my agenda: organize schedule of observations; find out about length of stay; behavioral expectations for residents; how they come here in the first place. TK said that my scheduling observation times were no problem, now that I'd met some people and he didn't hear any complaints. "I'm sure you have a non-threatening way with people" TK said (PC). Sudden shift of interest as TK says "I think there's something going on outside; excuse me" (PC) and quickly goes outside. When he left I took quick notes of the office: three desks and chairs, padlocked three drawer filing cabinet; yellow heavy drapes hung crookedly. He was back in less than one minute and said that he often has to chase drug dealers away from the building but they were running away when he got there. TK said he doesn't want them hassling or intimidating the residents. Same reason that back parking lot is fenced and locked immediately after cars drive in or out.

Asked TK about expectations and limits here for the residents. He explained that the "beauty of this kind of place . . . why I'm dressed in shorts, besides that it's comfortable . . . is that there is some structure, yet not enough to threaten people. I like to keep things casual" (PC). 'I may remind someone to shave or take a bath, but as long as they're not bothering anyone what they do is OK.' When I asked him what would be unacceptable, he said if they pushed the "outer limits" which included doing drugs or alcohol, selling either, or threatening others in the house. Another break in our conversation happened when TK got a call from his car dealer and DM (resident) came in to get his daily $2 and cigarettes. I said hello to him by name but he didn't make eye contact or respond verbally. [OC: was it the setting that put him off, me sitting in the office with a pen and notebook, or doesn't he remember me?]

TK off the phone and talking to me about the weekends, stating that there are fewer staff on weekends because residents don't have appointments and no resident-related calls to deal with. [OC: do family and friends use the weekends to visit?] Tom told me to introduce myself to Wesley, the handyman and deliverer of mail [OC: find out what else Wesley does; do residents ever help him? Are they allowed to?]

C:/Smythe/Research project AC-433/fieldnotes.doc

processing programs. It is important to write in the first person and differentiate your 'voice' from direct quotations or paraphrased material. Designating observer's comments (OC) about feelings, assumptions, concerns, fears and researcher-related issues by writing OC in the margins can be useful. Alternatively, such comments can be recorded in a separate fieldwork journal/research diary, which will be analyzed as part of the reflexive process. Writing field notes may take two to three times as long as the hours of participant observation, especially for novice researchers. This amount of time may seem daunting but, in our experience, the time passes quickly once the writing process is started, as recollections and interest in the observations take over.

Fieldwork journals and analytic diaries

There is considerable overlap in the content and purpose of fieldwork journals and analytic diaries. If both strategies are used, it is useful to differentiate the computer files (or notebooks) from one another so that emerging analytic ideas can be separated from more personal reflective writing. According to Spradley (1980) fieldwork journals 'will contain a record of experiences, ideas, fears, mistakes, confusions, breakthroughs, and problems that arise during fieldwork' (p. 71). This overlaps with the observer's comments that some researchers choose to write as field notes. Fieldwork journals or research diaries contribute to reflexivity, and thus data analysis, by providing a place for the researcher to explore thoughts and feelings about the research process.

An analytic diary is a format that a researcher uses to propose hunches and begin making connections among the data. Initially, it is written informally and leads to 'analytic memos' later. According to Hammersley & Atkinson (1995) 'the construction of analytic notes and memos therefore constitutes precisely the sort of internal dialogue, or thinking aloud, that is the essence of reflexive ethnography' (pp. 191–192). Analytic memos are also used in grounded theory studies and include a description of the codes used for analysis and identify the need for further theoretical sampling in order to test an emerging theory (Pope et al., 2006).

Documents

Official documents are one of the many 'unobtrusive' forms of data that supplement primary methods of data generation. These documents may be public, and range from archival policy records to codes of ethics, agency brochures and program descriptions, or they may belong to an organization and require permission to access (Bogdan & Biklen, 2003). Collection and analysis of these kinds of documents can function to triangulate data and enrich the analysis. If, for example, the research was focused on physical accessibility within a municipality and interviewing disabled people was the primary data generation method, it would be useful to examine city policy statements, proposals to city council from advocacy groups and newspaper articles. Other kinds of public documents are exemplified by written material that Suto (2000) analyzed in a board and care home. There was a facility description, schedules of activities and facility routines, announcements of events and a patient's bill of rights that all contributed to answering her research question about the environment, occupations and future-time perspective. There was a striking disjuncture between the written information and the actual environment. Hammersley & Atkinson (1995) caution researchers to critically analyze public and private documents and suggest the following questions:

- How are documents written?
- How are they read?
- Who writes them?
- Who reads them? For what purposes? On what occasions? With what outcomes?
- What is recorded? What is omitted?
- What does the writer seem to take for granted about the reader(s)?
- What do readers need to know in order to make sense of them? (p. 173)

Personal documents encompass a range of writings and are used by researchers to understand the participants' experiences, perspectives and actions through their own words (Bogdan & Biklen, 2003). Diaries, personal letters, email correspondence, writings on a particular topic and autobiographies constitute data that can be analyzed in various ways. Solicited accounts allow the participant to reveal things about herself or himself that may not arise in interviews or through participant observation (Hammersley & Atkinson, 1995). The participant may be uncomfortable discussing certain topics face to face or may find other forms of communication more effective. In Padilla's (2003) research with Clara, the data included Clara's 72 email messages interspersed with 11 face-to-face interviews. As Clara, who had sustained a traumatic brain injury 21 years prior to the study, explained: 'I prefer writing – speaking takes too much effort and control, and I find I lose concentration on the ideas when I try to also concentrate on controlling my body' (p. 415). McCuaig & Frank (1991) explored the adaptive patterns and choices made by a person – Meghan – with cerebral palsy in living an independent life. They used Meghan's personal documents as the most efficient means of communication, due to her inability to speak. In addition to participant observation and interviews using augmentative communication technology, Meghan shared her life story through typed diaries in response to McCuaig's questions and arduously produced over 150 pages of text. These two examples demonstrate how useful personal documents can be to generate data with some disabled people who might otherwise be excluded from research.

Other forms of data

Supplementary data may be generated through photographs, drawings, popular culture documents, such as films and television, and advertisements. The use of photography in qualitative research has its roots in nineteenth-century social documentaries of poverty in London by John Thomson and of New York City immigrants by Jacob Riis (Bogdan & Biklen, 2003). Photographs may be taken to document natural and built environments used by research participants and inter-actions within those settings, or collected for the same purpose. Baker & Wang (2006) adapted a participatory action research method called 'photovoice' to explore how pain experiences of older adults affected their social relationships. Particip-ants were instructed to take a photograph of an image that represented their pain and then photograph something that reflected a life without pain, and finally write brief narratives explaining the meaning of their photographs. Despite limita-tions and modifications to the method, Baker & Wang (2006) advocated further exploration and refinement of photovoice in health research. Guillemin's (2004) use of drawings to augment interview and survey data in studies of menopause and heart disease demonstrates another departure from word-based text. Although not yet well-represented in rehabilitation research, these forms of data generation may be appropriate for some research designs. Scanners provide the means to import non-text-based data such as photographs and drawings into computer-assisted ana-lysis of qualitative data (CAQDAS) and word processing programs.

Data management and computer applications

Qualitative researchers use computer software in varying degrees to assist with data management and subsequent analysis. The choice of which application to use is influenced partly by the research design, which includes the objectives, amount and type of data, the approach to analysis, the researcher's preferences, time and budget (Flick, 2006). An exploratory project with one researcher, few participants, a limited budget and text-based data may be effectively managed without buying specialized programs. Alternatively, some CAQDAS are designed to organize and assist in the analysis of video, photographic and acoustic media, something that exceeds the capabilities of word processing programs.

An evaluation of personal preferences and skills should also be made when decid-ing on qualitative research applications. The extent of the researcher's computer skills, interest in learning and time available to learn should be factored into the decision about which application to select. Some novice researchers may not want to learn a CAQDAS when they attempt their first project. The many features of CAQDAS may also prove distracting and leave little time or energy to make good decisions about managing and analyzing the data. The technical tasks of organ-izing and displaying data can be greatly enhanced by CAQDAS such as NVivo, ATLAS.ti and Ethnograph. Morse & Richards (2002) state that CAQDAS 'allow researchers not only to store materials but also to store ideas, concepts, issues, questions, models and theories' (p. 80). We recognize the advantages of these fea-tures but caution that there are no shortcuts to the intellectually demanding work of data analysis and interpretation, which are completed by the researcher, not by a computer program. In making decisions about computer applications to assist with storage and analysis, it is important first to identify the project needs and then determine which program provides the best fit. The rapid proliferation of CAQDAS applications and revisions preclude us from examining particular ones in any depth, as such a discussion would soon be dated.

Qualitative research applications, for example standard word processing, text retrieval and text-base manager, code-based theory building and conceptual networking programs, are categorized by the features they offer (Flick, 2006). Standard word processing programs allow the researcher to input data, edit, search for words, and create an unlimited number of files of coded chunks of data through a 'cut-and-paste' feature or macro commands. These programs require no learning or additional costs and may prevent the distraction of more complex applications. Seale (2000) discusses these features but states that CAQDAS complete tasks more quickly than word processing programs. He acknowledges, however, that word processing programs are more appropriate for small data sets.

Text retrieval and text-base manager programs typically feature searching, summarizing, listing and sorting functions, and order and administer data (Flick, 2006). The most popular programs are the code-and-retrieve sort that offer Boolean search functions, that is, the insertion of 'and', 'or' and 'not' to retrieve different data sets (Hesse-Biber & Leavy, 2006). Code-and-retrieve programs separate text for coding plus mark, order, sort and link texts and codes for later presentation. Code-based theory building programs incorporate code-and-retrieve program features and also 'allow the researcher to analyze the systematic relationships among the data, the codes, and code categories' (Hesse-Biber & Leavy, 2006, p. 361). Lastly, conceptual networking programs offer a high level of analytic assistance and graphically display networks of categories and potential new conceptual linkages (Flick, 2006). The features of these applications may be difficult to appreciate until the researcher begins to work with data rather than read about them. The CASDAQS Networking Project (2007) has established a useful website for current information, products and free demonstration copies of computer applications.

The question is whether to use a word processing program or purchase a CAQDAS appropriate for the research project. There is no doubt that CAQDAS can streamline certain aspects of data management and analysis. Alternatively, a word processing program can assist with taking notes in the field, writing field notes, editing text, coding, searching and retrieving, and writing memos and reports (Flick, 2006). Hesse-Biber & Crofts (cited in Hesse-Biber & Leavy, 2006) pose the following questions to help researchers think through their software program decision.

1. What type of computer do you prefer to work on or feel most comfortable working on? What excites you about this program at a visceral level?
2. Does the look and feel of the program resonate with your own research style?
3. How might each program enhance (or detract from) your analysis?
4. What research project or set of projects do you anticipate using a computer software program for?
5. How do you want a computer program to assist you?
6. What resources are available to you?
7. What are your preconceptions about these programs?
8. Which of the above questions/concerns are most important to you? (pp. 363–364)

Regardless of whether researchers choose a word processing program or a CAQ-DAS, it is essential that they become familiar with, in fact immersed in, the data. This familiarity occurs through reading and rereading interview transcripts, field notes and other data and transcribing the data. We return now to the topic of transcription and explore the benefits and drawbacks to using a transcriptionist.

Transcription

Employing a transcriptionist saves the researcher time that may be used for other research activities, such as ongoing data collection and analysis. Given that many rehabilitation research projects use interviews and focus groups as a primary data collection method and practitioner–researchers often have limited time allocated to research, transcriptionist services are desirable. Alternatively, a researcher who types quickly and has a transcription machine may prefer interacting with the data through the transcription process and content errors are less likely to occur, particularly when listening to interviewees who speak with different accents. Researchers adhering to a co-constructionist perspective of knowledge building may be more confident that they alone can identify the subtle nuances of speech production. There are also more subtle issues to consider when deciding to work with a transcriptionist.

Gregory *et al.* (1997) identify the vulnerability of individuals who transcribe interviews, especially if the content is disturbing and there are repeated interviews with the same research participants. They are concerned that transcriptionists are viewed as technical assistants and that little is done to prepare them for difficult interview material. MacLean *et al.* (2004) acknowledge those issues and propose that transcriptionists should be visible in the research process because they are 'participating consciously or not in a transforming auditory experience' (p. 118). That participation includes the use of 'emotional content notations' (p. 117) in which the transcriptionist tries to identify the speaker's feeling or intent by the way their speech sounds. A judicious use of these parenthetical notations and sufficient supervision is advised to reduce inaccurate interpretations by the transcriptionist. The view of transcriptionists as part of the research team lends credence to practices such as signed confidentiality agreements with the transcriptionist to protect the privacy of interviewees and research budgets that provide appropriate remuneration for their respected contributions. It is the researcher's responsibility to anticipate potential ethical issues related to religious beliefs or position in the community when using the services of a particular transcriptionist. When doing research in small communities or with some ethnocultural groups, it may be inappropriate for the transcriptionist to learn about the personal details and circumstances of research participants who are community members. Thus, the decision to use the services of a transcriptionist should be informed by examining the issues we have identified here.

In this chapter, we have presented practical ways of preparing and managing data and identified where there are links between the researcher's data management choices and subsequent analytic approaches. In the next chapter, we will discuss the reflexive and interpretive nature of the qualitative data analysis process and describe a foundational thematic approach to analysis.

References

Baker, T.A. & Wang, C.C. (2006) Photovoice: use of a participatory action research method to explore the chronic pain experience in older adults. *Qualitative Health Research*, *16* (10), 1405–1413.

Bird, C. (2005) How I stopped dreading and learned to love transcription. *Qualitative Inquiry*, *11* (2), 226–248.

Bogdan, R.C. & Biklen, S.K. (2003) Qualitative research for education: an introduction to theory and methods (4th edn). Boston, Allyn & Bacon.

Carpenter, C. (2004) Dilemmas of practice as experienced by physical therapists in rehabilitation settings. *Physiotherapy Canada*, *57* (1), 63–74.

CASDAQS Networking Project (2007) *Computer Assisted Qualitative Data Analysis Systems*. Retrieved 23 February 2007 from: http://caqdas.soc.surrey.ac.uk

Denzin, N.K. & Lincoln, Y.S. (2005) Introduction: the discipline and practice of qualitative research. In: N.K. Denzin & Y.S. Lincoln (eds), *The Sage Handbook of Qualitative Research* (3rd edn, pp. 1–32). Thousand Oaks, Calif., Sage.

Flick, U. (2006) *An Introduction to Qualitative Research*. London, Sage.

Green, J. & Thorogood, N. (2004) *Qualitative Methods for Health Research*. London, Sage.

Gregory, D., Russell, C.K. & Phillips, L.R. (1997) Beyond textual perfection: transcribers as vulnerable persons. *Qualitative Health Research*, *7*, 294–300.

Guillemin, M. (2004) Understanding illness: using drawings as a research method. *Qualitative Health Research*, *14* (2), 272–289.

Hammersley, M. & Atkinson, P. (1995) *Ethnography: Principles in Practice* (2nd edn). London, Routledge.

Hesse-Biber, S.N. & Leavy, P. (2006) *The Practice of Qualitative Research* (p. 56). Thousand Oaks, Calif., Sage.

Laliberte-Rudman, D. & Moll, S. (2001) In-depth interviewing. In: J.V. Cook (ed.), *Qualitative Research in Occupational Therapy: Strategies and Experiences* (pp. 24–51). Albany, NY, Thomson Learning.

Lofland, J., Snow, D., Anderson, L. & Lofland, L.H. (2006) *Analyzing Social Settings: a Guide to Qualitative Observation and Analysis* (4th edn). Belmont, Calif., Wadsworth/Thomson Learning.

McCuaig, M. & Frank, G. (1991) The able self: adaptive patterns and choices in independent living for a person with cerebral palsy. *American Journal of Occupational Therapy*, *45*, 224–234.

MacLean, L.M., Meyer, M. & Estable, A. (2004) Improving accuracy of transcripts in qualitative research. *Qualitative Health Research*, *14* (1), 113–123.

Mattingly, C. & Fleming, M.H. (1994) *Clinical Reasoning: Forms of Inquiry in a Therapeutic Practice*. Philadelphia, F.A. Davis.

Meadows, L.M., Lagendyk, L.E., Thurston, W.E. & Eisener, A.C. (2003) Balancing culture, ethics and methods in qualitative health research with Aboriginal peoples. *International Journal of Qualitative Methods*, *2* (4), Retrieved 3 January 2007 from: http://www.ualberta.ca/~iiqm/backissues/2_4/pdf/meadows.pdf

Morse, J.M. & Richards, L. (2002) *Read Me First for a User's Guide to Qualitative Methods.* Thousand Oaks, Calif., Sage.

Murphy, E. & Dingwall, R. (2003) *Qualitative Methods and Health Policy Research.* New York, Aldine De Gruyter.

Padilla, R. (2003) Clara: a phenomenology of disability. *American Journal of Occupational Therapy,* 57, 413–423.

Parry, R.H. (2006) Communication practices in physiotherapy: a conversation analytic study. In: L. Finlay & C. Ballinger (eds), *Qualitative Research for Allied Health Professionals: Challenging Choices.* Chichester, UK, John Wiley & Sons.

Pope, C., Ziebland, S. & Mays, N. (2006) Analysing qualitative data. In: C. Pope & N. Mays (eds), *Qualitative Research in Health Care* (3rd edn, pp. 63–81), London, BMJ Books.

Seale, C. (2000) Using computers to analyse qualitative data. In: D. Silverman (ed.), *Doing Qualitative Research: a Practical Handbook* (pp. 154–174). London, Sage.

Spradley, J.P. (1980) *Participant Observation.* New York, Holt, Rinehart & Winston.

Suto, M. (2000) Issues related to data collection. In: K.W. Hammell, C. Carpenter & I. Dyck (eds), *Using Qualitative Research: a Practical Introduction for Occupational and Physical Therapists* (pp. 35–46). Edinburgh, Churchill Livingstone.

Suto, M. & Frank, G. (1994) Future time perspective and daily occupations of persons with chronic schizophrenia in a board and care home. *American Journal of Occupational Therapy,* 48, 7–18.

Chapter 7
ANALYZING QUALITATIVE DATA

Introduction

Qualitative data analysis can seem the most complex and mysterious of all the phases of a qualitative project, partly because it receives the least thoughtful discussion and detailed description in the literature (Thorne, 2000; Sandelowski & Barroso, 2002). The language associated with qualitative analysis may vary depending on the methodological approach used by the researcher, and is often confusing and poorly defined (Dickie, 2003). Consequently, it is difficult to know what the researchers actually did during this phase and to understand how their findings evolved from the data (Thorne, 2000). In recognition of these criticisms, Dickie (2003) provides a detailed account of her analytic process that may prove illuminating to someone embarking on qualitative analysis for the first time. A description of the procedural details and nuances associated with the different methodology approaches is beyond the scope of this book. However, these approaches do share common theoretical assumptions that are represented in the basic interpretive thematic analytic approach that we will discuss in this chapter. We will also briefly highlight specific approaches associated with phenomenology and grounded theory and discuss the concept of reflexivity, which is of central importance to the qualitative analytic process. In recent years, qualitative researchers, influenced by the concept of evidence-based practice, have been engaged in a vigorous debate about the desirability and feasibility of combining qualitative findings or data by conducting a metasynthesis or meta-analysis and we will discuss this latest development in Chapter 10.

The analytic process

'Data analysis is the process of moving from raw interviews to evidence-based interpretations that are the foundation for published reports. Analysis entails classifying, comparing, weighing and combining material [obtained during data collection] to extract the meaning and implications, to reveal patterns, or to stitch together descriptions of events into a coherent narrative' (Rubin & Rubin, 2005, p. 201). Qualitative researchers tend not to be very explicit about their approach to data analysis or to define their use of the terms and concepts. The interpretive thematic analytic approach described in this chapter can be simply defined as 'a method for identifying, analyzing and reporting patterns (themes) within the data'

(Braun & Clarke, 2006). In our experience, this approach effectively provides those researchers new to qualitative research with core analytic skills that will be useful for conducting studies based on different traditions. Thematic analysis derives more from an ethnographic or grounded history tradition than phenomenology, but should be seen as a foundational approach to qualitative analysis. It is important, however, to recognize that the guidelines we provide in this chapter are exactly that – they are not rules or a recipe, and this basic analytic approach will need to be applied flexibly in specific studies to fit the research questions and data (Braun & Clarke, 2006).

As we have described earlier, the analytic process begins in the data acquisition phase during which decisions can be made to modify the design and pursue emerging ideas. Despite the fact 'that data collection is inescapably a selective process' (Miles & Huberman, 1994, p. 55), regardless of the purpose of the research or methodology employed, a qualitative approach frequently generates a daunting amount of data, usually in the form of words. The best defense against overload, according to Miles & Huberman (1994), is a well-thought-out research design, the focus of which is clearly established by the development of a conceptual framework and consistently articulated research question or purpose. The analytic process 'is a very time-consuming and labour intensive business' (Mason, 2002, p. 9) and a systematic approach to data organization and retrieval, as described in Chapter 6, is essential.

Qualitative analysis has been described as being in three phases: data reduction, data display, and conclusion drawing and verification (Miles & Huberman, 1994). *Data reduction* involves the researcher selecting, simplifying, abstracting and transforming the data that appear in written up field notes or transcripts. In this phase, the researcher makes analytic decisions – which data chunks might form categories, which to code and pull out, which patterns (or themes) best summarize a number of data chunks (or categories), and which evolving story to tell. At this stage, it may also be useful to generate simple frequencies, although these are usually considered to contribute only at the descriptive level of analysis. *Data display* is a key element of the analytical process. It can be achieved by physically organizing the data related to specific categories or codes in the same place; by producing diagrams, charts, matrices and maps of the main concepts; or by using the retrieval function of computer-assisted qualitative data analysis systems (CAQDAS) (Coffey & Atkinson, 1996). These diagrams may, or may not, actually be used in presenting the data to others. Their importance lies in the way they help the researcher to recognize patterns and relationships between data, which are difficult to see when data are in a text-based format (Mason, 2002). A lengthy text, for example the transcript of a 90-minute interview or focus group, is 'sequential rather than simultaneous, poorly structured, and extremely bulky' (Miles & Huberman, 1994, p. 11). Using such texts, researchers may be tempted to jump to hasty, unfounded conclusions and find only simplifying patterns. Throughout the research process, the qualitative analyst gains an increasingly in-depth understanding of the topic of interest by noting patterns, explanations and meanings, and identifying connections and relationships between data, the participant's context and theoretical concepts. The competent researcher, however, 'holds these conclusions lightly [and maintains] openness and skepticism' (Miles & Huberman, 1994, p. 11). It is during the third phase of *conclusion drawing and verification* that these conclusions or findings become explicit. The meanings emerging from the data have to be tested for their confirmability and credibility, for example by asking critical questions of the data, soliciting a peer review and ensuring that the participants 'voices' are fully represented. At this stage of the analysis the themes that have been discovered may be systematically related to form a coherent model or theory that explains a broader perspective or offers an explanation of why things occur the way they do (Rubin & Rubin, 2005). In this way, qualitative data analysis relies on inductive reasoning processes to interpret and structure the meanings that can be derived from the data (Thorne, 2000).

Miles & Huberman (1994) provide a straightforward and useful overview of the qualitative analytic process that we will now explore in more detail. Each researcher experiences this process differently. Sometimes it is isolating and frustrating, but often absorbing, intellectually stimulating and rewarding, and it involves numerous iterations, copious reflective memos and cups of tea (Dickie, 2003). The *data reduction* phase begins with reading and rereading the data. This reading can occur, as Mason (2002) suggests, 'at three different levels – literally, interpretively, and reflexively – and many qualitative researchers read on all three levels' (p. 149). A literal reading will provide information about the words and language used, the sequencing and structure of the interactions, and the literal content. While this information may prove useful if the focus of the research is purely descriptive, it is rare that qualitative analytic process will stop there. In reading the data interpretively, the researcher constructs and documents a unique version of what the data means and represents in relation to the research focus, and how the participants interpret and understand the phenomena of interest. It involves 'reading through and beyond the data' (Mason, 2002, p. 149) and is perhaps most synonymous with an exploratory research focus. A reflexive reading of the data seeks information about how the researcher is located in the data collection process and the role the researcher plays in generating and interpreting the data. An interpretive research focus would require a combination of all three levels of reading.

The data reduction phase requires researchers to immerse themselves in the data in order to organize, manage, abstract and retrieve the most meaningful sections of the data. This essentially means 'condensing the bulk of the data sets into analyzable units by creating categories with and from the data' (Coffey & Atkinson, 1996, p. 26). It begins by going through the transcripts (including field notes and documentary material) and highlighting *chunks of data* of varying size – words, phrases, sentences, or whole paragraphs – that appear to inform or provide insights about the research question or purpose. These data chunks can be highlighted by a variety of different methods, such as using coloured pens or a CAQDAS package. In determining the significance of these chunks of data, also called units of meaning or units of analysis, it is not the words themselves that are important but the meaning that matters. The choices about the significance of each chunk or fragment of data and the subsequent coding decisions are embedded in the researcher's prior understanding of the topic of interest and the conceptual framework developed in designing and implementing the research (Miles & Huberman, 1994).

The next phase of the analysis process is coding or indexing. Some authors (Mason, 2002; Pope & Mays, 2006) suggest that the term 'indexing' is more appropriate for use in qualitative research, as the term 'coding' is reminiscent of assigning numerical codes in a quantitative sense. However, coding is a central concept in the grounded theory approach and has been widely adopted by qualitative researchers. Codes are shorthand labels – usually a word, short phase, or metaphor – often derived from the participants' accounts, which are assigned to data fragments defined as having some common meaning or relationship. 'Coding thus links all those data fragments to a particular idea or concept' (Coffey & Atkinson, 1996, p. 27). Miles & Huberman (1994) suggest that coding represents the link between the raw data and the researcher's interpretive decisions by enabling the researcher to quickly find, pull out and cluster the data segments that relate to a particular construct, concept or theoretical idea. This coding process can be implemented in a variety of manual styles; for example margin keywords or code words can be assigned to highlighted data segments, and index cards can be used to cross reference instances to numbered pages, paragraphs or lines in the text. General cut-and-paste functions of word processing software or the data management function of CAQDAS programs also greatly facilitate coding and retrieving data, and clustering similarly coded data segments into categories. *Categories* can be defined as 'limited, concrete, and discrete entities that emerge most commonly from analysis of interview transcripts, observed events and documents' (DeSantis & Ugarriza, 2000, p. 239). Some categories can be represented by a single code, while others may overlap or intersect, and it is possible for the same data segment to have more than one code attached to it (Coffey & Atkinson, 1996). The question often asked is, 'How many categories should there be?' Mason (2002) suggests that problems arise in terms of analysis if too few or too many categories have been identified. If there are too few categories it may mean that there is inadequate data collection or that the coding is too broad or general. If there are too many categories it may mean that some are irrelevant or that they were refined or focused too early in the process. It may be useful in the category formation stage for the researcher to develop descriptions of each of the categories and associated codes outlining the ideas or concepts represented by them.

Miles & Huberman (1994) consider *displaying the data*, using concept maps, in preparation diagrams, matrices, taxonomies or tables, to be an integral component of determining overlap and linkages between categories for the next stage of the analytic process. 'Such displays are focused [distilled] enough to permit a viewing of a full data set in the same location, and are arranged systematically to answer the research questions at hand' (pp. 92–93). Written descriptions, analytic memos and data displays make the data more coherent and permit careful comparisons, detection of differences, and recognition of trends and patterns as well as contrast, paradoxes and irregularities. The exceptions, misfits and so-called negative findings should be seen as having as much importance to the analytic process as data that fit (Miles & Huberman, 1994; Coffey & Atkinson, 1996). During this process, codes, which are not carved in stone, can be abandoned and renamed and categories reformed and subsumed. In this phase the data are interrogated; for example the researcher could ask a question like, 'Are the categories fully representative of the participant's interpretations, events and settings?' In interpreting and theorizing the data, the researcher systematically moves between the concrete data and abstraction of the data, and brings to bear personal experience and knowledge of the literature and associated concepts in generating meaning or developing theory. The emerging categories are clustered or amalgamated together to form a smaller number of *themes* and represents a process of moving to higher levels of abstraction. Miles & Huberman (1994) describe a number of 'tactics for generating meaning' (p. 245), including clustering, making metaphors (for example referring to the empty-nest syndrome in relation to parents who have grown children), counting frequency of word use or the number of respondents making the same observations, comparing and contrasting data, subsuming the particular into the general and noting factors that contribute or intervene in relationships between variables (for example administrative support contributing to the relationship between standard of clinical practice and organizational change). Researchers typically do not explain how themes, which are reported as the main findings of a study, were derived from categories (Sandelowski & Barroso, 2002). Displaying the data, writing descriptions of categories and codes, and documenting tactics clearly can help provide the level of detail needed to track and make the analytic process transparent.

In a basic thematic interpretive approach, the *conclusion drawing and verification* phase consists of the development of a number of overarching themes. A theme can be defined as 'an abstract entity that brings together concepts, ideas or experiences, which often are meaningless when viewed alone' (DeSantis & Ugarriza, 2000, p. 359). 'As such, a theme captures and unifies the nature or basis of the experience into a meaningful whole' (p. 362). As DeSantis & Ugarriza (2000) point out:

> Presenting large numbers of themes . . . is equivalent to giving the reader unanalyzed, raw data and prevents any meaningful interpretation of findings. It is true that people may experience multiple themes simultaneously and that multiple themes do emerge from data, but the identification of large numbers of themes in any one study dilutes the unifying function of a theme (p. 368).

Because themes convey a sense of wholeness, overall patterns or repetition, they are derived from at least two and usually more categories, and are usually small in number. For example, Carpenter (2004) identified three major themes of dilemma experiences as described by physical therapists working in rehabilitation settings: justifying physical therapy knowledge in rehabilitation practice; the experience of moral distress in rehabilitation practice; and issues of interdisciplinary collaboration in rehabilitation. This extensive study involved multiple interviews with ten participants over a period of six months. Carpenter (2004), employing an interpretive data analysis approach, initially identified approximately 30 categories from which the three major themes eventually emerged. The questions related to developing themes frequently asked by researchers are: 'How prevalent should a theme be in the data?' 'What proportion of my data set needs to display evidence of a theme for it to be considered a theme?' 'How many themes should there be?' Of course, this being qualitative research there are no hard and fast concrete answers to these questions. Braun & Clarke (2006) offer the following advice in responding to these questions. It is not necessary for a theme to be present in an established percentage of the data, for example 50%, below which it would not be considered a theme. Equally, a theme does not need to be represented throughout the data set. A theme 'might be given considerable space in some data [chunks], and little or none in others, or it might appear in relatively little of the data set' (p. 82). The importance of 'a theme is not necessarily dependent on quantifiable measures – but rather on whether it captures something important in relation to the overall research question' (p. 82).

The language of 'emerging' themes, used extensively in the qualitative research literature, can be confusing as it conjures up the picture of thematic analysis as a passive process and 'denies the active role the researchers always plays in identifying patterns/themes, selecting which are of interest, and reporting them to the readers' (Braun & Clarke, 2006, p. 80). The description of themes 'emerging' or 'being discovered' can, as Ely *et al.* (1997) suggest 'be misinterpreted to mean that themes "reside" in the data, and if we look hard enough they will "emerge" like Venus on the half shell. If themes "reside" anywhere, they reside in our heads from our thinking about our data and creating links as we understand them' (pp. 205–256). The core issue is that this is an interpretive act on the part of the researcher and what is important is that researchers are consistent in how they engage in the analytic process and how they document it for others to understand.

The themes represent the findings of the study and it can be difficult to decide how best to write them up in a final report. It is unusual to find the prevalence of themes documented as a quantifiable measure. Descriptors like 'the majority of participants' or 'many participants' or 'a number of participants' are often used to convince the reader that the themes really existed in the data and that they are reporting their findings accurately (Braun & Clarke, 2006). However, as Braun & Clarke (2006) question, do such descriptors actually tell us anything? The way themes are presented depends on the research question and the type of analysis method being used. If a rich in-depth description is required then the reader needs to get a sense of the data as a whole and the themes should accurately reflect the entire data set. 'This might be particularly useful when . . . investigating an under-researched area or [if the researcher] is working with participants whose views on the topic are not known' (Braun & Clarke, 2006, p. 83). This type of analysis is more closely related to the questions asked during the data collection phase. In contrast, the analytic process could be guided more by the researcher's conceptual framework or preconceptions, an interest in individual motivations or understandings, or the desire to identify and examine the ideas, assumptions or ideologies that inform the data. According to Braun & Clark (2006), thematic analysis can be framed as an essentialist or realist approach in that it aims to report the 'experiences, meanings and the reality of participants' (p. 81), or it can be constructivist in nature and aim to 'examine the ways in which events, realities, meanings and experiences are the effects of a range of discourses operating within society' (p. 81) or a culture. In summary, thematic analysis is a flexible approach that is driven by the research question or purpose and the broader theoretical assumptions underpinning the research.

An illustration of thematic analysis

To illustrate the phases of qualitative thematic data analysis we have adapted data from a hypothetical study developed by our colleague, Dr Clare Taylor, for the purposes of teaching qualitative data analysis to occupational therapy and physical therapy students. The purpose of this study could be to explore the individual experience of panic attacks. In such a study, the data collection method would most likely be semi-structured interviews. The data provided represents ten different participants' responses to the question, 'Can you describe a typical panic attack for me?' The highlighted chunks of data (alternatively called units of meaning, units of analysis, or data fragments) appear to illuminate the topic or provide insights about the panic attack experience (see Table 7.1). The next stage is to code each of the data chunks (units of meaning) using a word or phrase in the transcript margin that appears to represent the meaning in the statement

Table 7.1 Identifying meaning data 'chunks' or 'fragments'.

Participant	
#1	Actually, I don't think there is any such thing as a typical panic attack. **They are all different, which is what makes them so scary . . . the unpredictability of them!** I find them so difficult to handle – the not knowing. **Sometimes I think I can predict what will set me off, but I can't really. I hate the uncertainty. I hate them!**
#2	**Breathing into a paper bag helps,** but I have no idea why! So I always carry a paper bag whenever I go out. **Sometimes being outside brings on an attack,** but not always, so I can't stay home all the time can I? That's no way to live . . . so when I feel myself winding up **I try using the bag.** It does seem to help calm me down if I catch it quickly enough.
#3	**I go hot and cold, start to sweat** and just want to run out of the room. **I start to breathe very quickly. I worry about what I might do,** whether I am going to faint. **I just have to escape to a quiet place.** Then I try to talk myself through it and tell myself that I can cope, that I'm not dying, and that I will be able to calm down and finish what I was doing.
#4	**They always happen to me when I am traveling.** I love traveling, but I get myself into a state. I worry that I've lost the tickets, that I'll miss the train or the flight or whatever. **It's dreadful if I get stuck in a queue.** Then **I start to sweat. I go all cold and clammy, my breathing gets very fast.** So I start to **do the relaxation things my therapists taught me.** I tell myself

Table 7.1 (cont'd)

Participant	
	that I haven't forgotten anything. I go through all the positive statements and things. They usually work, but it can take a few minutes and it feels like forever.
#5	**There's no such thing as a typical attack, let me tell you. Sometimes I sweat, sometimes I can't concentrate, sometimes I think I'm going to faint and the world goes black around the edges.** But they all seem to be different. I do sometimes wonder if **I'm going to have a heart attack.** It feels just like my Dad described his [heart attack] but I'm never sure how they are going to take me . . . it's hard.
#6	Well, I've only had one, or maybe two . . . what I call, real panic attacks. The one I can really remember happened in a supermarket. I was shopping and **I just came over all hot and I couldn't catch my breath.** I thought there was something really wrong, and I just had to get outside and take lots of breaths, you know almost gulping . . . That's the only thing I think of as a panic attack . . . I get nervous and worried if I have to talk to people I don't know but I don't think of that as a panic attack.
#7	Oh, **being in a dark room especially at night** . . . that will do it, bring one on. I have to sleep with the curtains open. **I can't stand feeling closed in, and I must have the window open,** otherwise **I get hot and sweating and I feel like I can't breathe** and **I have to find a way out.** I have to find a window and open it, then I can breathe fresh air. **I'm hopeless in air-conditioned rooms** that don't have any windows you can open – really hopeless!
#8	Well, **they're all so different!** I keep trying to see if there is a common something, but sometimes **I'm in shop or meeting, once I was on a bus** and I've even started feeling a bit odd when I'm in the house or office on my own . . . **it's frightening. I get shaky and feel like I might faint or have a heart attack, and the edges of what I see go all black . . . and I breathe fast,** someone said to **breathe into a paper bag,** but I haven't tried that, well not yet anyway . . . do you think it does any good?
#9	**Traveling, that does it. I had to stop traveling on the Tube. I can't cope with all that darkness.** I was down there once, we were stuck in a tunnel and it was so hot, **I couldn't escape. I was cold and hot and clammy . . . I thought I was going to faint or throw up** or do something **to disgrace myself.** I couldn't cope with that. **I'd be embarrassed.** Anyway, this young lass next to me, oh, she was ever so sweet, she looked after me, **she talked to me and sort of calmed me down** and told me to **breathe into a paper bag** if it happened again. But I just stopped traveling on the Tube. I suppose I should go to the doctor about it, but it seems so silly.
#10	I used to panic ever such a lot when I was a student. **I would get into such a state before exams, or even handing essays in. I couldn't concentrate.** I thought I was going mad, **I just wanted to run away.** Sometimes **I'd get a tight chest, I couldn't breathe and I thought I was having a heart attack.** But then I saw someone, and **I learnt to relax and to think positively.** It's helped me manage the panicky feelings and I don't get into such a state now.

(see Table 7.2). In the next phase of the analytic process, the coded data is abstracted from each participant's transcript. Commonalties and linkages between the categories are sought and negative cases are identified for further exploration in subsequent data collection. A clear data management strategy, as described in Chapter 6, is essential in order that data, for example participants' quotes, can be easily tracked to the original source. At this stage it may be useful to display

Table 7.2 Indexing or assigning codes to the data.

Participant	Data	Code
#1	Actually, **I don't think there is any such thing as a typical panic attack.** They are all different which is what makes them so scary . . . **the unpredictability of them! I find them so difficult to handle – the not knowing. Sometimes I think I can predict what will set me off but I can't really. I hate the uncertainty.** **I hate them!**	All different Emotional response Uncertainty Uncertainty Uncertainty Emotional response
#2	**Breathing into a paper bag helps,** but I have no idea why! So **I always carry a paper bag whenever I go out. Sometimes being outside brings on an attack,** but not always, so I can't stay home all the time can I? That's no way to live . . . so when I feel myself winding up **I try using the bag.** It does seem to help calm me down if I catch it quickly enough.	Strategy Strategy Trigger Strategy
#3	**I go hot and cold, start to sweat** and just want to run out of the room. **I start to breathe very quickly. I worry about what I might do,** whether I am going to faint. **I just have to escape to a quiet place.** Then **I try to talk myself through it and tell myself that I can cope,** that I'm not dying, and that I will be able to calm down and finish what I was doing.	Symptoms Symptoms Emotional response Strategy Strategy
#4	**They always happen to me when I am traveling. I love traveling, but I get myself into a state.** I worry that I've lost the tickets, that I'll miss the train or the flight or whatever. **It's dreadful if I get stuck in a queue.** Then **I start to sweat. I go all cold and clammy, my breathing gets very fast.** So I start to **do the relaxation things my therapists taught me.** I tell myself that I haven't forgotten anything. **I go through all the positive statements and things.** They usually work, but it can take a few minutes and it feels like forever.	Trigger Related to location Symptom Strategy Strategy
#5	**There's no such thing as a typical attack, let me tell you. Sometimes I sweat, sometimes I can't concentrate, sometimes I think I'm going to faint and the world goes black around the edges. But they all seem to be different.** I do sometimes wonder if **I'm going to have a heart attack.** It feels just like my Dad described his [heart attack] but I'm never sure how they are going to take me . . . it's hard.	All different Symptoms All different Symptoms

Table 7.2 (cont'd)

Participant	Data	Code
#6	Well, I've only had one, or maybe two . . . what I call, real panic attacks. The one I can really remember happened in a supermarket. **I was shopping** and **I just came over all hot and I couldn't catch my breath.** I thought there was something really wrong, and I just had to get outside and take lots of breaths, you know almost gulping . . . That's the only thing I think of as a panic attack . . . I get nervous and worried if I have to talk to people I don't know but I don't think of that as a panic attack.	Related to location Symptoms
#7	Oh, **being in a dark room especially at night** . . . that will do it, bring one on. **I have to sleep with the curtains open.** I can't stand feeling closed in, and **I must have the window open,** otherwise **I get hot and sweating and I feel like I can't breathe** and **I have to find a way out. I have to find a window and open it,** then I can breathe fresh air. **I'm hopeless in air-conditioned rooms that don't have any windows you can open** – really hopeless!	Related to location Trigger Strategy Symptom Strategy Strategy Trigger
#8	Well, **they're all so different,** I keep trying to see if there is a common something, but sometimes **I'm in shop or meeting, once I was on a bus** and I've even started feeling a bit odd when I'm in the house or office on my own . . . **it's frightening. I get shaky and feel like I might faint or have a heart attack, and the edges of what I see go all black . . . and I breathe fast,** someone said to **breathe into a paper bag,** but I haven't tried that, well not yet anyway . . . do you think it does any good?	All different Related to location Emotional response Symptoms Strategy
#9	**Traveling, that does it. I had to stop traveling on the Tube. I can't cope with all that darkness.** I was down there once, **we were stuck in a tunnel** and it was so hot, **I couldn't escape. I was cold and hot and clammy . . . I thought I was going to faint or throw up or do something to disgrace myself. I couldn't cope with that. I'd be embarrassed.** Anyway, this young lass next to me, oh, she was ever so sweet, she looked after me, **she talked to me and sort of calmed me down** and told me to **breathe into a paper bag** if it happened again. But I just stopped traveling on the Tube. I suppose I should go to the doctor about it, but it seems so silly.	Trigger Trigger Trigger Symptoms Emotional response Emotional response Strategy Strategy
#10	I used to panic ever such a lot when I was a student. **I would get into such a state before exams, or even handing essays in. I couldn't concentrate.** I thought I was going mad, **I just wanted to run away.** Sometimes **I'd get a tight chest, I couldn't breathe** and I thought I was having a heart attack. But then I saw someone, and **I learnt to relax and to think positively.** It's helped me manage the panicky feelings and I don't get into such a state now.	Trigger Symptoms Strategy Symptoms Strategy

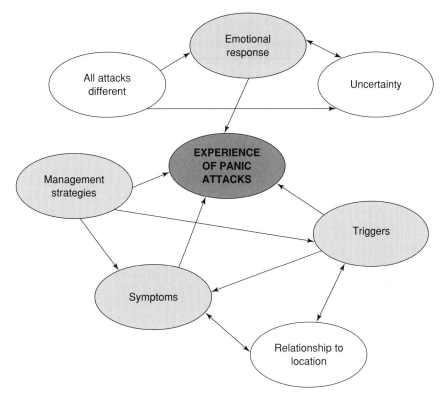

Figure 7.1 Displaying the data.

the data, for example by constructing manual or computer diagrams, charts or maps (see Figure 7.1), or physically sorting coded data using cards or wall displays. Displaying the data may help to identify where connections or relationships within the data exist and assist in reducing the data by amalgamating or integrating categories into a smaller number of themes. In our simple illustration you can see that the category coded 'related to location' overlapped with 'symptoms' and 'triggers', and the decision was made to subsume it with the category 'triggers' to become a theme with that name. Similarly, specific 'management strategies' were related to offsetting the effects of the 'triggers'. The categories coded as 'all attacks different' and 'uncertainty' overlap with 'emotional response' and were integrated to form one theme. This interpretive process is guided by the established purpose of the study and so questions used to interrogate the data focus on understanding the experience of panic attacks. In this hypothetical example the themes, presented in Table 7.3, have been generated from the responses to only *one* question and, as such, represent preliminary findings only. They could be revised and reinterpreted as the data analysis progressed to encompass data generated from the full interviews. Comprehensive descriptions of the themes could be produced and supported by appropriate data examples. Graphical representation and, on occasion, frequencies can assist in illustrating the analytic decisions and findings.

Table 7.3 Presenting the themes.

Themes	Frequency	Illustrative quotes
Symptoms		
• Sweating/hot and cold	60%	I start to sweat. I go all cold and clammy (R4)
• Breathing problems	40%	I couldn't catch my breath (R6)
• Feeling faint/fear of fainting	40%	I think I'm going to faint and the world goes black around the edges (R5)
• Tight chest/thoughts of heart attack	30%	I thought I might faint or have a heart attack (R8)
• Loss of concentration	20%	I couldn't concentrate (R10)
• Need to escape	20%	I couldn't escape (R9)
		I wanted to run away (R10)
Management strategies		
• Controlling breathing	50%	Breathing into a paper bag helps (R2)
• Escaping/fresh air/ changing location	30%	I just have to escape to a quiet place (R3)
		I have to find a window and open it (R5)
• Relaxation techniques/ calming	30%	I start doing the relaxation things that my therapist taught me (R4)
• Positive thinking	30%	I learnt to relax and to think positively (R10)
		I talk to myself and tell myself I can cope (R3)
Triggers		
• Being outside/amongst people	20%	Sometimes being outside brings on an attack (R2)
• Traveling	20%	The one I really remember happened in a supermarket. I was shopping (R6)
• Enclosed spaces/darkness	20%	They always happen to me when I am traveling. I love traveling, but I get myself into a state (R4)
• Stressful situations	10%	I had to stop traveling on the Tube. I can't cope with all that darkness (R9)
		I'm hopeless in air-conditioned rooms that don't have any windows you can open (R7)
		I would get into such a state before exams or even handing in essays (R10)
Emotional response to uncertainty		
• All different/uncertainty)	30%	The unpredictability of them! I find them so difficult to handle – the not knowing (R1)
• Frightening/scary	20%	It's frightening (R8)
• Worry/embarrassment	20%	They are all different which is what makes them so scary (R1)
• Anger	10%	I worry about what I might do (R3)
		I thought I would do something to disgrace myself. I couldn't cope with that. I'd be embarrassed (R9)
		I hate the uncertainty. I hate them! (R1)

The thematic analysis process we have described is a complex intellectual one through which the knowledge and experience of the participants is juxtaposed with the knowledge, sensitizing concepts and experience of the researcher. It is essential that researchers are clear about what they are doing and why, and include a thorough description of how they did their analysis in their written reports. 'Writing is an integral part of the qualitative analysis process, not something that takes place at the end, as it does with statistical analyses' (Braun & Clarke, 2006, p. 86). It begins during the data collection phases, continues throughout the study, provides additional data, and facilitates reflexivity. As Braun & Clarke (2006) emphasize, 'if we do not know how people went about analyzing the data, or what assumptions informed their analysis, it is difficult to evaluate their research, and to compare and/or synthesize it with other studies on that topic, and it can impede other researchers carrying out related projects in the future' (p. 80).

Reflexivity

The outcome of qualitative research is clearly a joint interpretive enterprise in which both parties work together to generate the research findings (Hammell & Carpenter, 2000). The researcher is an integral part of this process, articulating the research problem or purpose, shaping the collection of data and interpreting, explaining or describing human behavior from the perspectives of those participating in the study. This central role makes it impossible for the qualitative researcher to present an objective, dispassionate, distanced, non-contested account of other individuals' experiences. It is unrealistic to consider the elimination of the researcher as a person from the research process. For many of us newly engaging in qualitative research, this shift from the ideal of scientific detachment and controlling 'bias' to subjective interpretation is perhaps the most difficult to comprehend. The term 'bias' is associated with the idea that there is a single objective reality, and that it is possible to know that reality outside oneself (Jongbloed, 2000). In general, qualitative researchers recognize the relative, multiple and socially constructed nature of reality and how meanings are negotiated in particular contexts (Denzin & Lincoln, 2005). If multiple interpretations of the same event are assumed then the term 'bias' is misplaced in the context of qualitative research. The concept of reflexivity is a response to the concern with 'bias'.

Reflexivity is an essential strategy that enhances the quality of research by making explicit the deep-seated views and judgments that affect the research topic, including a full assessment of the influence of the researcher's background, perceptions and interests on the research process. It requires the researcher to systematically reflect on and analyze all aspects of the research design and implementation. Field notes, analytic memos and reflective journals are three approaches to constructing a reflexive account that addresses issues that we will discuss in more depth in the remainder of this chapter, namely, choosing the research question, the researcher's position, interaction with participants, reciprocity, managing self and representation.

Our interest in a problem, question or topic may be triggered by experiences or incidences at work or in our private lives, for example inequalities of service provision for clients with HIV/AIDS, or the experience of a disabled family member, or problems finding services for a child with learning disabilities. It is important to understand how the conceptualization and design of the research are situated in our professional or personal lives and how the data can affect us personally (Primeau, 2003). The concept of *positionality* is related to where one 'chooses' to speak. It involves the recognition that, as researchers, we speak from our perspective as members of a particular sex, gender identity, class, ethnic group, religion or profession (Carpenter & Hammell, 2000). These memberships are the lenses through which we view data collection and analysis. For example, Primeau (2003) described the importance of reflexivity in helping her to understand how her personal identification as an occupational therapist and feminist influenced her study. These perspectives shape our orientations, attitudes, values and interests and frame our research. They can contribute to the authenticity or credibility of the researcher and ground and direct the study process, shaping what we look for and see, as well as what we do not look for or see. Without conscientious reflection, these perspectives can limit our ability to be open to the meanings of others or to grasp the complexity of situations and experiences.

The interaction between researcher and participants is key to the data collection process and is influenced by how the researcher is perceived by the participants, for example as an expert, as someone who can be trusted or as someone who will provide advice. These perceptions are related to expectations and the concept of *reciprocity*. As Primeau (2003) suggests, people who tolerate a known observer or an interviewer in their life have every reason to ask, 'What do I get in return?' (p. 12). Most often, the trade-off is some type of assistance, a genuine interest in or validation of their experiences. These interactions need careful monitoring and negotiation if expectations and assumptions of both parties are not to cause confusion or conflict. Carpenter (2000) found that the individuals who were initially interviewed in her study exploring the experience of spinal cord injury became almost angry when asked open-ended questions characteristic of qualitative research. They expressed their discomfort by asking questions, such as: 'Am I telling you what you want?' 'What information do you need exactly?' 'What are you trying to get at?' All the participants knew of the researcher's connection, as a physical therapist with the rehabilitation center, and it became clear that they had made assumptions about the nature and purpose of the interview based on their experience of being interviewed by therapists in the rehabilitation setting, when questions were predictable and focused on acquiring specific information. The concept of reciprocity, which implies give and take, and a mutual negotiation of meaning and power in the research process, is central to discussions about conducting ethical and responsible qualitative research. Reciprocity requires, on the part of the researcher, a genuine presence, self-disclosure and commitment to involving participants in all phases of the research.

Researchers may find themselves unexpectedly emotionally involved during the course of their interactions with participants, for example feeling grief, shock or revulsion in response to something they hear or observe, or differing values and assumptions may become evident during data collection. Finlay (1998), who explored 'the life world of occupational therapists', experienced anger on behalf of a patient and frustration at one occupational therapist's inability to communicate more assertively with doctors on behalf of the patient. Self-reflection led her to interpret her own responses and locate what appeared to be the main issues underpinning what she was observing and hearing.

Coffey (1999) suggests that researchers cannot control how stakeholders in the research process, such as participants, professional colleagues or gatekeepers, perceive their participation. However, in reality, researchers create different self-presentations for different settings, and engage in a process of impression management while in the field, and these strategies need to be acknowledged and recorded in terms of how they shape the data. Arber (2006) provides a detailed reflexive accounting of her dual identity as a practitioner and a researcher within an ethnographic study in the context of a hospice. She identifies the dynamic nature of presenting herself as requiring constant work and monitoring of oneself and the reactions of others. At different times, she presented herself as a mother, nurse practitioner or nurse researcher, as approachable, non-threatening, non-intrusive, friendly, empathetic, animated, interested, engaged or agreeable as specific situations required, and she consistently monitored her non-verbal responses during her interactions with the stakeholders involved in the study. Primeau (2003) describes how she found herself 'in the throes of a dilemma with which ethnographers are typically faced, that is, how to simultaneously strive for connection and rapport with the participants and yet minimize [her] intrusiveness and the inevitable effects of [her] presence on [the participants'] daily life experiences' (p. 13). As she goes on to describe, 'my field notes are peppered with reflexive accounts of the ways in which I tried to avoid participating in the very events that I was there to observe' (p. 13).

Qualitative research is often conducted by members of a group or professional affiliation, or a related affiliation, such as a practitioner conducting research with clients, rather than by complete strangers. Carpenter (2004), a physical therapist, conducted research to explore dilemmas of rehabilitation practice as experienced by members of her own profession. This insider status meant that she shared a common reality and language that facilitated the interview dialogue and enabled her to probe for deeper understanding and meaning. It also, however, meant that she brought to the research certain assumptions and opinions about rehabilitation practice which shaped the data collection and analysis processes. There may be particular issues for practitioners, such as therapists or nurses, as they negotiate a research relationship rather than a therapeutic relationship. Kuhl (2002), a general practitioner and palliative care physician, conducted a phenomenological study to explore what it meant to live with a terminal illness such as cancer or AIDS. He describes how he had to learn to listen in a different way, set aside the biases inherent in the physician approach to terminal illness, to stop seeking to predict, explain, or control the disease's progression. With each participant, he had to renegotiate the relationship, focusing on their expertise and his role as a learner rather than as a physician.

Reflexivity is a central concept and closely related to the ethical issues that are characteristic of qualitative research. A reflexive approach means that researchers should interrogate their own beliefs and feelings in the same way that they will interrogate those of the participants. Thus, at all stages of the research, the impact of the researcher in terms of access to data, relationships in the field, and how one is identified as the researcher, as a practitioner or both should be documented and become part of the analysis process. Reflexivity is not an open invitation to bare our souls or make us, as researchers, the focus of the research report. It should, however, provide those who read the report with enough detail to enable them to make a judgment about how and where the researcher influenced the research collection, analysis and dissemination of the findings.

Alternative approaches to data analysis

In Chapter 4, we discussed a number of influential qualitative methodological approaches, in particular phenomenology and grounded theory, for which detailed and sophisticated data analysis procedures have been developed. We highlight some of the important features of these analytic processes in this chapter and recommend some useful references for those who wish to explore these further. Phenomenological approaches seek the structure or essence of human experience through intensive study of individual cases. Thorne (2000) provides this example to illustrate the focus of phenomenological analysis. A phenomenological study:

> Rather than explain the stages and transitions within grieving that are common to people in various circumstances, ... might attempt to uncover and describe the essential nature of grieving and represent it in such a manner that a person who had not grieved might begin to appreciate the phenomenon (p. 69).

The analytic approach therefore orients the researcher to an exhaustive, reflective and detailed analysis of each individual experience. A number of phenomenologists (for example Colaizzi, 1978; Giorgi & Giorgi, 2003; Smith & Osbourne, 2003) have developed structured frameworks that assist with the complex analysis of phenomenological data. In Chapter 4, we introduced bracketing or *epoche* as being an important concept in phenomenology. Phenomenological approaches characteristically challenge the researcher to set aside or bracket all preconceptions about the phenomenon in order that they can work inductively to generate new insights and understanding about individual experience. Bracketing should not be confused with an attempt to be 'objective'; on the contrary, it requires that researchers reflect intensively on their own experiences, values and beliefs about the phenomenon of interest. Sanders (2003) provides a useful description of how she applied Colaizzi's (1978) framework to the analysis of data from a phenomenological exploration of spirituality, and Reynolds (2003) examines Smith & Osbourne's (2003) interpretative phenomenological approach to analyzing the data from a study exploring the reasons women give for engaging in artistic occupation as a means of coping with illness.

As we discussed in Chapter 4, the key features of grounded theory focus on analytic strategies rather than sampling or data collection (Charmaz, 2000). This approach offers considerable structure and is characterized by being cyclical and iterative, that is, from the beginning of the research, the processes of collecting, coding and analyzing data are conducted at the same time. Data collection is guided by theoretical sampling. The point of theoretical sampling is to select sources of new data in ways that permit the further development of theory. Theoretical sampling involves the ongoing inclusion of additional individuals, groups, situations and settings. These sampling decisions inform and are informed by successive revisions of the emerging theory. This represents a major component of the constant comparative method, which is at the heart of grounded theory. Glaser & Strauss (1967) refer to integrating categories and their properties as the other important component. Through a process of coding, briefly described in Chapter 4, a set of categories is generated from the initial comparison of data. These categories can then be compared and clarified through analysis of newly acquired data. This process leads to the formulation of theory that is solidified through reduction. In using the term reduction, Glaser & Strauss (1967) meant that the researcher 'may discover underlying uniformities in the original set of categories or their properties, and can then formulate the theory with a smaller set of higher level concepts' (p. 110). Reduction enables categories to be expressed at a greater level of abstraction and therefore generality. With the acquisition of new data, it becomes clear whether existing categories are theoretically saturated and therefore no further coding is required, or whether the new data requires existing codes or categories to be modified. Glaser & Strauss are the main proponents of grounded theory, but since their first seminal book, published in 1967, they have adopted differing perspectives, particularly towards the data analysis process. An in-depth discussion of the intricacies of the complex and structured data analysis process they have collaboratively (Glaser & Strauss, 1967) and separately developed (Glaser, 1992; Strauss & Corbin, 1998) is beyond the scope of this book. Bluff (2005) provides a useful overview of the application of grounded theory in health care and, like us, she encourages researchers who are interested in undertaking a grounded theory study to make explicit the approach they have adopted.

In this chapter we have attempted to clarify, without oversimplifying, the basic principles and concepts associated with qualitative data analysis. The qualitative analytic process is by definition a flexible, interpretive and creative one and, as such, can be difficult for researchers new to qualitative research to come to grips with. In this chapter, we have been particularly careful to make explicit the terminology we chose to use, as the diverse vocabulary associated with qualitative research and lack of clarity in published research accounts can also be confusing. We provided an illustration of a basic thematic analysis that can be viewed as foundational to more sophisticated approaches developed in grounded theory and phenomenology. In the next chapter, we move from data collection and analysis to discuss issues related to dissemination of qualitative findings.

References

Arber, A. (2006) Reflexivity: a challenge for the researcher as practitioner? *Journal of Research in Nursing*, 11 (2), 147–157.

Bluff, R. (2005) Grounded theory: the methodology. In: I. Holloway (ed.), *Qualitative Research in Health Care* (pp. 147–167). Oxford, Blackwell.

Braun, V. & Clarke, V. (2006) Using thematic analysis in psychology. *Qualitative Research in Psychology*, 3, 77–101.

Carpenter, C. (2000) Exploring the lived experience of disability. In: K.W. Hammell, C. Carpenter & I. Dyck (eds), *Using Qualitative Research: a Practical Introduction for Occupational and Physical Therapists* (pp. 23–33). Edinburgh, Churchill Livingstone.

Carpenter, C. (2004) Dilemmas of practice as experienced by physical therapists in rehabilitation settings. *Physiotherapy Canada*, 57 (1), 63–74.

Carpenter, C. & Hammell, K.W. (2000) Evaluating qualitative research. In: K.W. Hammell, C. Carpenter & I. Dyck (eds), *Using Qualitative Research: a Practical Introduction for Occupational and Physical Therapists* (pp. 107–119). Edinburgh, Churchill Livingstone.

Charmaz, K. (2000) Grounded theory: objectivist and constructivist methods. In: N.K. Denzin & Y.S. Lincoln (eds), *Handbook of Qualitative Research* (2nd edn, pp. 509–535). Thousand Oaks, Calif., Sage.

Coffey, A. (1999) *The Ethnographic Self*. London, Sage.

Coffey, A. & Atkinson, P. (1996) *Making Sense of Qualitative Data*. Thousand Oaks, Calif., Sage.

Colaizzi, P.F. (1978) Psychological research as the phenomenologist views it. In: R.S. Valle & M. King, (eds), *Existential Phenomenological Alternatives for Psychology* (pp. 48–71). New York, Oxford University Press.

Denzin, N.K. & Lincoln, Y.S. (eds) (2005) Introduction: the discipline and practice of qualitative research. In: N.K. Denzin & Y.S. Lincoln (eds), *The Sage Handbook of Qualitative Research* (3rd edn, pp. 1–32). Thousand Oaks, Calif., Sage.

DeSantis, L. & Ugarriza, D.N. (2000) The concept of theme as used in qualitative nursing research. *Western Journal of Nursing Research*, 22 (3), 351–372.

Dickie, V.A. (2003) Data analysis in qualitative research: a plea for sharing the magic and the effort. *American Journal of Occupational Therapy*, 57 (1), 49–56.

Ely, M., Vinz, R., Downing, M. & Anzul, M. (1997) *On Writing Qualitative Research: Living by Words*. Oxford, Routledge/Farmer.

Finlay, L. (1998) Reflexivity: an essential component for all research? *British Journal of Occupational Therapy*, 61 (10), 453–456.

Giorgi, A.P. & Giorgi, B.M. (2003) The descriptive phenomenological psychological method. In: P.M. Camic, J.E. Rhodes & L. Yardley (eds), *Qualitative Research in Psychology: Expanding Perspectives in Methodology and Design* (pp. 243–271). Washington, DC, American Psychological Association.

Glaser, B.G. (1992) *Basics of Grounded Theory Analysis: Emergence vs Forced*. Mill Valley, Calif., Sociology Press.

Glaser, B.G. & Strauss, A.L. (1967) *The Discovery of Grounded Theory: Strategies for Qualitative Research*. Chicago, Aldine.

Hammell, K.W. & Carpenter, C. (2000) Introduction to qualitative research in occupational therapy and physical therapy. In: K.W. Hammell, C. Carpenter & I. Dyck (eds), *Using Qualitative Research: a Practical Introduction for Occupational and Physical Therapists* (pp. 1–12). Edinburgh, Churchill Livingstone.

Jongbloed, L. (2000) Choosing the methodology to explore the research. In: K.W. Hammell, C. Carpenter & I. Dyck (eds), *Using Qualitative Research: a Practical Introduction for Occupational and Physical Therapists* (pp. 13–21). Edinburgh, Churchill Livingstone.

Kuhl, D. (2002) *What Dying People Want: Practical Wisdom at the End of Life*. Toronto, Doubleday Canada.

Mason, J. (2002) *Qualitative Researching* (2nd edn). London, Sage.

Miles, M.B. & Huberman, A.M. (1994) *Qualitative Data Analysis* (2nd edn). Thousand Oaks, Calif., Sage.

Pope, C. & Mays, N. (eds) (2006) *Qualitative Research in Health Care* (3rd edn). London, BMJ Books.

Primeau, L.A. (2003) Reflections on self in qualitative research: stories of family. *American Journal of Occupational Therapy*, 57 (1), 9–16.

Reynolds, F. (2003) Exploring the meanings of artistic occupation for women living with chronic illness: a comparison of template and interpretive phenomenological approaches to analysis. *British Journal of Occupational Therapy*, 66 (12), 551–558.

Rubin, H.J. & Rubin, I.S. (2005) *Qualitative Interviewing: the Art of Hearing Data* (2nd edn). Thousand Oaks, Calif., Sage.

Sandelowski, M. & Barroso, J. (2002) Finding the findings in qualitative studies. *Journal of Nursing Scholarship*, 34 (3), 213–219.

Sanders, C. (2003) Application of Colaizzi's method: interpretation of an auditable decision trail by a novice researcher. *Contemporary Nurse*, 14, 292–302.

Smith, J.A. & Osbourne, M. (2003) Interpretative phenomenological analysis. In: J.A. Smith (ed.), *Qualitative Psychology: a Practical Guide to Research Methods*. London, Sage.

Strauss, A. & Corbin, J. (1998) *Basics of Qualitative Research: Techniques and Procedures for Developing Grounded Theory*. Thousand Oaks, Calif., Sage.

Thorne, S. (2000) Data analysis in qualitative research. *Evidence Based Nursing*, 3 (3), 68–70.

Chapter 8
WRITING AND DISSEMINATING QUALITATIVE RESEARCH

Introduction

In this chapter, we explore the process through which the researcher moves from analyzing and interpreting the data, to presenting and discussing the evidence or research findings. Essentially, the writing process articulates the outcome of data analysis – what has been discovered, what it means, its implications and its level of contribution to professional knowledge. We will discuss important features that are integrated within this writing process, such as data selection, provision of a thorough audit or decision trail, faithful inclusion of the participant's perspectives and attention to representation of the participants. We will make the case that it is the researcher's responsibility to ensure that subsequent articles and professional presentations accurately represent participants' perspectives, are accessible for them to read and will benefit them. This chapter concludes with an overview of manuscript preparation and the peer-review process.

In preparation for writing the research report, it is important to identify its primary purpose and determine the parties to whom the researcher is accountable and responsible. Clarity of one's position on these issues guides the decisions that the researcher needs to make about what findings to present, who constitutes the audience and where to publish. This thinking process may also reveal tensions that exist for the researcher between producing research that is consistent with a client-centered philosophy and reproducing knowledge that is acceptable to rehabilitation professionals but does not challenge the role that rehabilitation practitioners play in disabled peoples' lives (Hammell, 2006). Writing and disseminating research are neither neutral nor apolitical activities; rather, they form part of the grounded commitments that influence a researcher's decision about who and what concerns are worthy of research (Frank, 1997).

Why are you writing? – What is your objective?

The research and subsequent publications will normally contribute to rehabilitation sciences in one or more of the following ways: provide evidence to support practice, advance conceptual development, aid in program planning, or evaluate programs. An understanding of the 'utilization value' (Smaling, 2003, p. 20) of reported research findings can encourage researchers to be more accountable for clearly identifying their research findings, demonstrating how they enhance previous knowledge and applying them to specific practice settings. Sandelowski (2004) suggests a utilization framework in which research use can be classified as instrumental, symbolic and conceptual as a means of understanding, demonstrating and enhancing how qualitative research findings can be used to generate new knowledge. *Instrumental utilization* 'is the concrete application to practice of research findings that have been translated into material forms, such as clinical guidelines, care standards, appraisal tools, care pathways and intervention protocols' (Sandelowski, 2004, p. 1371). Schachter *et al.* (2004) reported on the development of a practitioners' handbook on sensitive practice that exemplifies the practical (instrumental utilization) application of qualitative research. In addition to publishing their research in physiotherapy and social work journals, these researchers effectively translated their knowledge into a resource for academic and practice environments. In contrast, according to Sandelowski (2004), '*symbolic utilization* is less visible and concrete, as it entails no change per se, but rather the use of research findings as a persuasive tool to legitimate a position or practice' (p. 1371). The findings from studies about experiences of enjoyment for people with schizophrenia constitute less tangible (symbolic utilization) but equally important contributions to evidence (Laliberte-Rudman *et al.*, 2000). Research findings that advance *conceptual development* also comprise evidence for practice, but this kind of research utilization 'is the least tangible . . . as it entails no observable action at all, but rather a change in the way users think about problems, persons or events' (Sandelowski, 2004, p. 1371). The value of conceptual findings is to promote understanding through interaction with knowledge, recognizing that understanding and thinking differently about people and their lives are indeed actions, albeit difficult ones to discern. Within rehabilitation, conceptual development abounds, with some researchers producing modest explanatory models such as Rebeiro & Cook's (1999) occupational spin-off and participation in mothering tasks processes (Backman *et al.*, 2007). Through their research about the nature of clinical expertise, Gwyer *et al.* (2004) produced a theoretical model that illuminated the key dimensions and processes of expert practice. This research has the potential to change how practitioners develop and frame opportunities for student learning. Another form of conceptual development results when researchers work with existing concepts, as McCuaig & Frank (1991) did with adaptation and independent living, to illuminate the personal and contextual features that create an 'able self'. Despite qualitative research presenting an uncomfortable fit on occasion, Sandelowski (2004) argues that it offers an important corrective to 'the scientific aesthetic of averages and dispassionate objectivity' (p. 1369).

The potential is great but there are few qualitative research reports that support program planning in physical therapy and occupational therapy. Rebeiro's (2004) dissatisfaction with the lack of evidence to support the use of occupation in mental health occupational therapy led her to complete a series of projects. The occupational spin-off model cited earlier, and other collaborative research projects that Rebeiro conducted with clients, supported the development of an alternative mental health program, with occupation as its central core (Rebeiro *et al.*, 2001). Rebeiro's body of research shows clearly that she writes for the benefit of mental health clients and her objective is to change occupational therapy practice.

Qualitative program evaluation is used to identify issues in a particular context, obtain an insider perspective from service users and assess the efficacy of services delivered (Galvin, 2005). The credibility of findings is enhanced by service users and providers' agreement about the process of evaluation. Participants need to be willing to accept unflattering findings that may, for example, have negative implications for future funding. When writing a report that uses qualitative research methodology to evaluate service delivery, the audience and objective of the report is clarified at the beginning of the project. Carpenter & Forman (2004) describe how focus groups were used in the qualitative phase of research that examined the efficacy of programs offered by a disability advocacy organization. In addition to supporting timely modifications to existing programs, the report generated useful findings for more successful collaboration between the advocacy organization, clients and rehabilitation service providers.

Research is incomplete until it has been written up and published in peer-reviewed journals and other formats where knowledge is disseminated. We write to have our work read, critiqued and ultimately used to change practice, inform policy and foster future research, in short 'to risk making a difference' (Unruh, 2007, p. 67). To fulfill this ideal, it is necessary to recognize one's responsibility to various research stakeholders: disabled people, rehabilitation professions, funding agencies, health boards and communities.

To whom are you responsible? What are the constraints and opportunities?

The dissemination of research findings begins with identifying the roles that individuals and organizations played in the study. Researchers receive financial support through scholarships from professional associations, health research funding agencies, universities and advocacy groups. Employers can offer reduced workloads to enable practitioners adequate time to conduct research without loss of income. The proportion of support received from these groups influences the order of priority and style of the reports produced. If an advocacy group funds the research, for example, the researcher may commit to writing reports for the organization and its membership before publishing in peer-reviewed journals. Program evaluation research findings are usually time sensitive and require quick dissemination, in various forms, to the parties involved. Participatory action research involves multiple stakeholders and the collaboration inherent in this type of inquiry continues through to the dissemination of findings (Letts, 2003).

Academic researchers, who often have research funded, are expected to publish in peer-reviewed professional journals and rehabilitation publications that reach a wider audience. Research graduate students are supported either directly through grants, or indirectly by their universities and thesis supervisors, and are encouraged to disseminate their findings in peer-reviewed journals. This point is especially relevant to students whose work forms part of their supervisor's over-all research endeavor and warrants co-authored publications. Participants play a pivotal role in research, but their goodwill has not always resulted in having the findings communicated to them; neither have they seen the benefits of such knowledge (Hammell, 2006). This practice is changing through the efforts of disability theorists and some rehabilitation researchers (for example Rebeiro, 2004; Hammell, 2006). Ultimately, researchers must determine the nature of their responsibility to those who have contributed to the project and establish the priority of subsequent publications to respect the support received.

Several questions arise as researchers think through how they will fulfill their responsibility to disseminate the research findings. Answers to these questions pro-vide guidance for writing the report and reveal the political nature of research. Who is the audience for the report? What is the purpose of communicating the findings? Where will the findings be published and how does this affect the writing style? The question least often asked is: 'Who will benefit from these publications?' The audience for a qualitative research report ranges from the research supervisor to government health and social services departments. The audience for reports to various levels of government, such as community health boards, can include bureaucrats and health professionals outside rehabilitation. Silverman (2000) outlines four audiences who have different expectations of research reports. The lay public is interested in learning about different ways to manage a chronic care condition, obtaining facts that may influence policy and confirming their own experiences. Practitioners expect theoretical advances but also know-ledge that can be translated to enhance service delivery. Policy makers are inter-ested in findings that are useful for justifying health care policies that institute or reduce services. Academic rehabilitation specialists are interested in theoretical advances applicable to research and practice education, factual knowledge and methodological insights.

Much of rehabilitation research is aimed at allied health care professionals. The primary audience is usually the researcher's own profession, whereas academics and practitioners in other health disciplines form the secondary audience. Re-searchers who write for professional audiences can assume some understanding of well-established social science and rehabilitation concepts, such as adaptation, recovery and stigma. This assumption should not be made for lay audiences, such as clients and their family members, who may be unfamiliar with these types of concepts and often more interested in the practical application of the findings.

The research utilization framework (Sandelowski, 2004), introduced earlier, offers a broad brushstroke to clarify the purposes of communicating research findings. These purposes vary across researchers and projects, and research findings from one project may achieve different aims depending on how they are presented. Researchers can write to persuade others of new perspectives that may contribute to professional education and/or challenge current practices. They can write to fulfill commitments to disabled people and contribute to interdisciplinary liter-ature, albeit in different publications. Rarely does one achieve all these purposes with one project, although Hammell (2000a, 2000b, 2003, 2004a) provides an example of how a number of publications gave her the opportunity to disseminate the complex findings derived from her quality of life research with people who live with high spinal cord injuries to different reader groups.

Writing for peer-reviewed professional journals requires selecting the appropriate journal for the research findings and using a formal, persuasive style. There is a high level of reading comprehension, a specific knowledge base and an expectation that the research report is original work that advances theory or practice involved in submitting a manuscript to this type of journal. Traditionally, research reports published in peer-reviewed journals were written in the third person, an influence from the positivist stance of quantitative research. More style variation is now found in physical therapy and occupational therapy journals, such as the selective use of the first person voice in qualitative research reports. The sections of an article typically include an introduction, a literature review, methodology, results/findings, discussion and a conclusion/summary. We discuss the submission and editorial process for peer-reviewed journals later in this chapter.

In contrast to professional journals, many lay publications target a variety of audiences with diverse reading and educational levels, and offer greater flexibility of writing styles and presentation formats. These kinds of publications expect knowledge to be translated appropriately for their audiences but do not normally want explication of discipline-specific theoretical constructs. While we support knowledge translation that benefits the people who contribute to the research we also recognize that the nature of some research is theoretical and may have little direct application to disabled people and other participants. In the next section, we introduce the concerns about 'who benefits from research?' and encourage researchers to consider this issue in relation to their own projects.

Nowhere do the complexities of dissemination of the research findings become more apparent than in disability theorists' critiques of accountability, that is, who benefits from research (Barnes *et al.*, 1999; Mercer, 2002). These critiques raise concerns about whose interest is being served with dissemination of findings and, indeed, the research endeavor itself. Mercer (2002) proposes that 'disability research should be judged in terms of its capacity to facilitate the empowerment of disabled people' (p. 245). The emancipatory disability paradigm from which these critiques arise uncovers a tension for rehabilitation researchers – fulfilling their discipline-specific professional responsibility versus being accountable to disabled people who are often research participants (Hammell, 2006). It is difficult to hear criticism that researchers have advanced their own careers by indirectly exploiting disabled people, doing little to change their lives in the process. It is true, however, that students earn degrees by doing research and academics use research findings to present at conferences, write papers and attract graduate students, all in the quest for promotion and funding. Thus, we agree with Hammell (2006) who contests the notion that research is necessarily altruistic and calls for a 'congruence between client-centered philosophy and research' (p. 168). Researchers can demonstrate their 'client-centerdness' by returning the research findings in accessible forms to the people who have been researched. Then, people have the choice to use this knowledge to suit their purposes such as influencing policy and gaining more control over their lives. Hammell (2006) argues that researchers make political choices that reflect their values when they decide how they write, what theories they draw on, where they choose to disseminate research findings, and in what formats. We believe that it is reasonable to examine what rehabilitation research has done for disabled people as well as the formats and locations in which the findings appear. Yet it is unrealistic to expect that all research should address the needs articulated by disability studies scholars and activists. Theory-driven rehabilitation research, for example, makes an impact in education and practice and is necessary to advance knowledge within the professions (for example Hammell, 2004b; Suto, 2004; Mortenson & Dyck, 2006).

How do you go about writing?

The aim of writing up qualitative research is to present a persuasive and engaging story, one that has a particular purpose and structure that differentiates it from journalistic reporting or creative writing. Among the main differences are the coherence of the research design, the purposive nature of the inquiry and the expectation that qualitative research findings will advance theory and practice (Morse & Richards, 2002). The purpose of writing is to illuminate the research process and, in doing so, provide readers with a cogent argument and sufficient detail to support the interpretation of the findings. Sandelowski (2004) proposes that the structure of qualitative reports should make the findings clearly distinguishable from other aspects of the research process, such as supporting literature, data and analytic procedures. Such clarity increases the likelihood that practitioners can evaluate the evidence and choose whether to incorporate it into their practice. This style of qualitative research writing is customary in peer-reviewed rehabilitation journals and addresses the evidence needs of rehabilitation practitioners. In contrast, representation styles, such as poems and plays that reflect post-modernist sensibilities, may be engaging and insightful but are generally less convincing as evidence useful for practice.

Writing the research report begins in earnest when the data analysis is completed and the findings can be articulated. This final step in the research process can be exciting but also somewhat daunting for novice researchers who might have difficulty getting started. One strategy that can help researchers start writing and reduce the expectation that the report must be perfect is to think of it as a draft (Bogdan & Biklen, 2003). It is important to write in a manner that respects the proposed audience, to craft sentences in such a way that a balance is struck between highly academic writing that is often inaccessible to a wide readership and simplistic writing that cannot do justice to complex concepts. Unruh (2007) and Murray (2004) offer practical resources for successful writing that are based on feedback solicited from experienced and novice writers about the habits and strategies that helped them write a paper for publication. These authors emphasize the importance of getting started, developing a writing routine and using the purpose of the research to guide the development of a paper structured by judicious use of headings. The following section makes some suggestions about headings that might be used and the type of content that might be included in a research report.

Introduction

The development of an outline is essential for deciding what to include in the report and organizing the content according to the requirements of the academic program or peer-reviewed journal (Unruh, 2007). An outline can also be helpful in determining which quotations will be used and where tables, figures or graphics should be placed. The introduction should present a timely and compelling problem, describe the purpose of the research and in this way encourage the reader to continue. The introduction sets up the problem by providing some background information that includes the larger context in which the study is situated. In Mortenson & Dyck's (2006) introduction, they briefly summarized the state of client-centered practice in occupational therapy and proposed that exploring day-to-day power relations at a systems level could illuminate the disconnection between therapists' principles and their practices. The purpose of their study was articulated in the introduction; alternatively, the purpose of the research question may be stated at the end of the background or literature review.

Literature review or background

The literature review or background section of a report provides a detailed account of research and conceptual literature that demonstrates the author's understanding of current knowledge. In this section, research studies, usually no older than 10 years, are critically reviewed to identify their strengths and weaknesses and to build a strong rationale for the study. A judicious use of older classic studies is acceptable, as are relevant conceptual writings and policy documents. For example, Heah *et al.* (2007) framed the background to their study by drawing on Canadian child health and social development databases and the person-environment-occupation model. They combined this knowledge with a review of empirical studies of children with disabilities and created an argument for their research, which sought to understand what motivated disabled children to participate in various activities and what role their disability played in participation. Quantitative and qualitative studies from within and outside rehabilitation disciplines may be reviewed to justify the research. Although an initial literature review occurs in the research design phase, it is advisable to update this review at the time of report writing, as several months (or even years) may have passed since the project's inception.

Research design

The research design section (alternatively called methodology or methods section) describes the process of the research: the theoretical framework (methodology), methods of generating data, approach to analysis, participant recruitment strategies, trustworthiness or integrity of the findings and reflexivity. In keeping with the flexibility of the research design and the interpretive nature of qualitative inquiry, this section requires a different kind of explication from the relatively brief description of research protocols that are appropriate for quantitative reports. The methodology needs to be explained in enough detail for the reader to have sufficient information upon which to judge its fit with the research question and the plausibility of the findings (Carpenter & Hammell, 2000; Dickie, 2003). Thus, a description of which theoretical frameworks were used and how they informed the researcher's thinking is far more useful than the cursory comments that sometimes appear in this section. Among the less illuminating statements are simply, 'I used a grounded theory methodology' or 'the study used qualitative methods', followed by citations of general qualitative research texts rather than specific and relevant publications that reflect the researcher's in-depth understanding of specific theoretical frameworks (Dickie, 2003). Teram *et al.* (2005) offer a good example of writing about methodological theories, specifically combining grounded theory with PAR, and explain the implications these choices had on the research.

The description of methods should address all the strategies that were used, for example interviews, participant observation and documentary materials, including those that were less successful at obtaining data than anticipated, such as self-reported time use logs or reflective journals (Suto, 2000; Carpenter, 2004). If interviewing was the method of choice, then explain how the interviews were structured, who conducted them, the average duration and the number of participants interviewed. For example, clarify whether the data are based on single interviews of each participant or repeated interviews over a particular time span. It is useful to provide a sample of the interview questions either within the article as a table, or as an appendix. The environment in which the interviews (or other data generation) occurred should be noted, as well as how the information was recorded and transcribed. For student research, it may be useful to indicate the kind of training or supervision received for the methods used. For research that involves clients, it is important to indicate whether the individual who conducted the interviews was also responsible for providing direct services to those clients as this may raise some ethical issues that need to be addressed.

A discussion of participant recruitment informs the reader about who was involved in the study, the criteria by which they were chosen and the sampling strategy that was used. When providing demographic information, which can be summarized in a table, select the important characteristics about the participants and avoid details that are irrelevant to the study, for example 'race', or identifying details that increase the likelihood of anonymity being compromised. Most journals require a statement indicating that the researcher has received ethical approval for the study from an academic or health authority institutional review board (IRB), or an equivalent community-based organization, and that participants have given informed consent.

Writing about the data analysis can be challenging as it requires the researcher to describe key elements of a complex cognitive process well enough to convince the reader that the interpretation of the data is plausible. This contributes to the audit or decision trail and details how the participants were involved after the data generation, for example reviewing transcripts or offering feedback about themes and interpretive frameworks. The trustworthiness of the findings may be enhanced by the confirmation of coding schemes and the review of selected transcripts by co-researchers. Howie *et al.* (2004) present an example of how coding transcript data was further abstracted to thematic categories, thus giving the reader a sense of the analytic process.

Information about the data analysis is most useful, however, when the discussion extends beyond descriptions of coding techniques and member checking to the presentation of significant turning points in the research process (Dickie, 2003). Dickie contends that a discussion about the questions that the researcher has grappled with can illuminate the data analysis process. Thus, answering the question, 'What aspects of the data became the puzzle, and how did the pieces finally fit together?' (Dickie, 2003, p. 52) assists the reader to understand how particular discoveries in the data supported or changed the researcher's thinking about the phenomena. Research journals, analytic memos and field notes help to reconstruct the twists and turns in the research process, and are used to create a reflexive account.

An examination of the researcher's presentation of self, interactions with participants and other features of reflexivity (described in Chapter 7), if written well, offers the reader additional information by which to judge the authenticity of the findings. Primeau (2003) demonstrates how field notes can contribute to reflecting on and writing about the impact that the researcher has on the research process. It is important to consider how the issues related to positionality influence the research and how power relations impact on the quality of the data. Were participants reluctant to criticize rehabilitation services because of your professional role? Were participants indirectly trying to limit their involvement by canceling interviews and having little time to reschedule them? Sometimes professional values and socialization can make it difficult to recognize how the views we bring to research may affect the data and subsequently, the findings. Two examples are offered to illustrate how a reflexive account might be constructed.

In her research, which used a life history approach, McCuaig (McCuaig & Frank, 1991) reveals that her unexamined optimism about what disabled people could achieve initially skewed the way she wrote about the participant. Through dialogue with her thesis advisor (Frank), McCuaig comes to understand how this perspective affected the presentation of data. She (McCuaig & Frank, 1991) describes the insight she gained as follows:

> In the course of developing a relationship with Meghan, the researcher had inadvertently denied the tension and the distress, the enormous effort, the vulnerability, and the tedium of living with a disability, and the effort required to carry out commonplace activities (p. 231).

In writing about this insight, McCuaig opens the door for readers to reflect on how their own beliefs and perspectives may influence research with disabled people. A reflexive excerpt from Padilla's (2003) phenomenological report uncovers how ableist ideology can permeate deeply held professional beliefs to shape the researcher's views and expectations:

> I began this project conscious that what attracted me to Clara in the first place was a sense of her heroism – that I had, in fact, been confronted with my ableist attitude the night I met her and rushed to keep her upright and later feigned understanding of her words. I recognized that I had been surprised by her perceptivity that evening and her eloquence in her first email message – that I too had a preconscious expectation that the appearance of her body was a representation of her mind. Yet, having recognized that, I still subconsciously set out on a 'heroic' path of my own – to research Clara's experience and give her the voice I erroneously presumed she did not have because of her difficulty with speech. (p. 420)

The ability and willingness of McCuaig and Padilla to explore their respective roles in the research suggests a depth of analysis that lends additional credence to the findings. Padilla's (2003) detailed description of the data analysis, including Clara's involvement, offers more insight into his thinking than is usual in published reports. In this way, the data analysis constitutes an essential link to the results or findings section of the report.

Findings/results

The aim of this section of a paper is to describe the research findings in such a way that the participants' words and the researcher's interpretive voice are both represented. *Representation* is an ethical concern and researchers have a duty to portray participants' experiences and opinions accurately and reflect the context in which the data were generated. There is an art to presenting findings that remain faithful to participants' perspectives and interpret their meaning. The findings answer the research question, whether they are presented thematically or at a higher conceptual level. Published qualitative research offers many examples of how to present findings. Typically, the researcher describes each theme and uses selected quotations from participants to support the credibility of themes. Quoted material requires careful editing to remove extraneous material while retaining the meaning (Morse & Richards, 2002). For example, utterances (uhms, ahs) and redundancies should be removed and occasional words can be inserted for clarity, the latter indicated by brackets. The use of ellipses is a standard practice that indicates where text has been removed within a single conversation. Quotations that are contextualized for the reader are more useful than free-standing text and short quotations can be a most powerful complement to the researcher's interpretive voice. The use of participants' words ensures an accurate representation of their unique perspectives and the expressive qualities as the researcher originally heard them.

The presentation of the findings reflects the methodological theory that guided the study. Thus, the explication of a social process based on a core category is required when grounded theory is used. With ethnography, the findings comprise an in-depth description of a cultural unit that illuminates customary practices, beliefs and understandings. When writing up the results, the use of pseudonyms may be insufficient to protect participant's anonymity and the location of the research setting. Therefore, it is acceptable to change details or present demographic data in aggregate form so that people and places cannot be identified. The contextualized nature of qualitative data and the credibility of the findings can be maintained by carefully revising or removing non-vital information.

Discussion

The researcher discusses the findings by incorporating relevant literature and examining practice models and theoretical constructs to position the new knowledge in a broader context. This is an opportunity to show how these particular findings add to an understanding about a concept or identify therapeutic practices that may, or may not, be helpful for clients and their families. In DeGrace's (2004) study, which addressed the question, 'How does a family with a child with autism negotiate the occupations of being a family?' (p. 544), she used the themes 'feeling robbed' and 'occupy and pacify' to show how autism pervaded the family unit, affecting its identity, development and integrity. This knowledge is relevant to therapists, who may use a family-centered model in their work but may be unaware of how their suggested interventions can impact on the whole family; that is, effective strategies for managing behavioral outbursts and keeping the autistic child occupied may leave little time or energy for activities that encourage family cohesiveness.

One way to structure the discussion section is to address each theme individually, as Howie *et al.* (2004) did, working with the literature to frame and integrate the findings. Depending on the objectives of the study, the researcher can use a practice model to extend or identify inadequacies revealed by the findings. Alternatively, the findings can be interpreted and discussed for different user groups such as clients, therapists, service providers and policy makers. The audience for DeGrace's (2004) research, for example, is most likely to be therapists working with autistic children, whereas Mortenson & Dyck's (2006) study is aimed at a broader audience of occupational therapy practitioners, educators and service providers. Depending on the publication, the implications of the research may be presented in this section or as part of the conclusion.

Conclusion

The conclusion may be a succinct paragraph or two that summarizes the intent and findings of the study. It may also include a discussion of the study limitations, ideas for future research and how the findings inform practice, theory or education, if these have not been discussed elsewhere. An explanation of what the study contributes should be included and such statements should be fully supported by the findings. There are always limitations and these should be noted without apologies. When writing about future directions for research, it is useful to pose the questions that need to be pursued next and suggest how they can best be answered. Acknowledgements are placed at the end of a report and convey appreciation to the participants who made the study possible, research mentors and others who have contributed to the study or reviewed the manuscript. Most journals follow the practice of indicating which studies were completed as partial fulfillment of a master's or doctoral degree. Agencies that funded the research are also named and acknowledged in this section.

How do you disseminate qualitative research?

Writing for publication in peer-reviewed journals requires an understanding of manuscript preparation and the editorial review process. Physical therapy and occupational therapy research is published in journals that are specific to each profession (for example *Physical Therapy*); have a health research mandate (for example *Qualitative Health Research*); focus on a particular practice area (for example *Psychiatric Rehabilitation Journal*); and address multiple rehabilitation issues (for example *Archives of Physical Medicine and Rehabilitation*). Familiarity with these kinds of journals can help authors choose the most appropriate one for their manuscript. Successful manuscript preparation depends on an understanding and adherence to author guidelines, which are published electronically or in print. These guidelines outline the content and style requirements to be followed. Although the quality of the report is the primary criterion for acceptance, good writers will edit their papers to ensure that they conform to the journal's maximum page length, required referencing system and other style expectations. It is important to review the manuscript using the published journal criteria and proofread it carefully for spelling and grammatical errors. To ensure that writing clarity has been achieved it is a good idea to ask a colleague who is a skilled writer but unfamiliar with the topic area to review the work and provide feedback.

Authorship is straightforward if there is only one researcher. In the case of co-researchers, it is advisable to determine the extent of each person's contribution to the research and decide who is responsible for writing all or parts of the report. This decision is made before submitting the report for publication and the order of names is based on the extent of each person's contribution, that is, the person who did the majority of the research and write-up is the first author. It is customary for each person who makes a substantial contribution to some aspect of the project – its conceptualization, the data gathering, analysis and/or writing the report – to be listed as an author on the manuscript. Student research and manuscript submissions customarily list the student as first author, but these are often strengthened by the contribution of their thesis supervisor, through actual writing, editing or general guidance. These student–supervisor research and publication relationships may be problematic, however, owing to the inherent power imbalance between the two parties and poor communication. Universities have policies that are designed to protect students and clarify issues such as first authorship when the student has been responsible for the majority of the work. We encourage students to seek out and use the appropriate academic process to communicate with their supervisors about future publications well before the writing commences. Despite the policies and procedures that exist, it may be difficult for some students to initiate this discussion and assert their rights in these situations.

Qualitative research report manuscripts are submitted to the editor of a peer-reviewed journal and undergo a systematic editorial process to determine their suitability for publication. Peers are volunteer review board members who are appointed by the editor and evaluate manuscripts that are within their areas of content and/or methodological expertise. Editors ensure that reviewers are blind to the author's identity. Suitability is based on several criteria, such as originality, quality of research design and credibility of findings, and writing ability. Manuscripts could have all of these qualities but be declined by the editor with a recommendation to submit to a different, more appropriate journal. Peer-review functions to ensure that manuscripts accepted for publication meet certain quality standards, will be of interest to readers and contribute knowledge that is either specific to physical therapy or occupational therapy, or to rehabilitation more generally. Reviewers aim to offer an unbiased, constructive critique of a manuscript, identifying areas of strength and focusing on weaknesses that necessitate revision if the paper is to be published. It is not unusual for a manuscript to be returned to the author with a request for revisions to be made before it is accepted for publication. The time between acceptance and appearance in the journal varies among publications but may be up to one year. Answers to these kinds of publication and peer-review questions can be found either in the journal or by contacting the editor.

While there are alternative ways of disseminating qualitative research, such as presentations (see Chapter 3), or creating web-based resources, we have focused in this chapter on providing practical guidance for writing research reports, particularly for publication in peer-reviewed journals. Researchers have a responsibility to facilitate translation or transfer of the knowledge generated as a result of their research and producing written accounts is a primary method of addressing the issue of knowledge translation. We will discuss this topic further in the next chapter as it relates to the use of evaluative criteria and strategies to ensure the trustworthiness and credibility of qualitative research.

References

Backman, C.L., Del-Fabro Smith, L., Smith, S., Montie, P.L. & Suto, M. (2007) The experiences of mothers living with inflammatory arthritis. *Arthritis and Rheumatism (Arthritis Care & Research)*, 57, 381–388.

Barnes, C., Mercer, G. & Shakespeare, T. (1999) *Exploring Disability: a Sociological Introduction*. Cambridge, Polity Press.

Bogdan, R.C. & Biklen, S.K. (2003) *Qualitative Research for Education: an Introduction to Theory and Methods* (4th edn). Boston, Allyn & Bacon.

Carpenter, C. (2004). Dilemmas of practice as experienced by physical therapists in rehabilitation settings. *Physiotherapy Canada*, 57 (1): 63–74.

Carpenter, C. & Forman, B. (2004) Provision of community programs for clients with spinal cord injury: using qualitative research to evaluate the role of the British Columbia Paraplegic Association. *Topics in Spinal Cord Injury Rehabilitation*, 9, 57–72.

Carpenter, C. & Hammell, K.W. (2000) Evaluating qualitative research. In: K.W. Hammell, C. Carpenter & I. Dyck (eds), *Using Qualitative Research: a Practical Introduction for Occupational and Physical Therapists* (pp. 107–119). Edinburgh, Churchill Livingstone.

DeGrace, B.W. (2004) The everyday occupation of families with children with autism. *American Journal of Occupational Therapy*, 58, 543–550.

Dickie, V.A. (2003) Data analysis in qualitative research: a plea for sharing the magic and the effort. *American Journal of Occupational Therapy*, 57, 49–56.

Frank, G. (1997) Is there life after categories? Reflexivity in qualitative research. *Occupational Therapy Journal of Research*, 17, 84–98.

Galvin, K. (2005) Navigating a qualitative course in programme evaluation. In: I. Holloway (ed.), *Qualitative Research in Health Care* (pp. 229–249). Oxford, Open University Press.

Gwyer, J., Jensen, G., Hack, L. & Shepard, K. (2004) Using a multiple case-study research design to develop an understanding of clinical expertise in physical therapy. In: K.W. Hammell & C. Carpenter (eds), *Qualitative Research in Evidence-based Rehabilitation* (pp. 103–115). Edinburgh, Churchill Livingstone.

Hammell, K.W. (2000a) Living from the neck up: society and high quadriplegia. *New Mobility*, 11 (79), 53–56.

Hammell, K.W. (2000b) High-level injury: self-managed care and quality of life. *Total Access* (Canadian Paraplegic Association), 1 (3), 31–32.

Hammell, K.W. (2003) Changing institutional environments to enable occupation among people with severe physical impairments. In: L. Letts, P. Rigby & D. Stewart (eds), *Using Environments to Enable Occupational Performance* (pp. 35–53). Thorofare, NJ, Slack.

Hammell, K.W. (2004a) Quality of life among people with high spinal cord injury living in the community. *Spinal Cord*, 42, 607–620.

Hammell, K.W. (2004b) Using qualitative evidence to inform theories of occupation. In: K.W. Hammell & C. Carpenter (eds), *Qualitative Research in Evidence-based Rehabilitation* (pp. 14–26). Edinburgh, Churchill Livingstone.

Hammell, K.W. (2006) *Perspectives on Disability: Contesting Assumptions, Challenging Practice*. Edinburgh, Churchill Livingstone Elsevier.

Heah, T., Case, T., McGuire, B. & Law, M. (2007) Successful participation: the lived experience among children with disabilities. *Canadian Journal of Occupational Therapy*, 74, 38–47.

Howie, L., Coulter, M. & Feldman, S. (2004) Crafting the self: older persons' narratives on occupational identity. *American Journal of Occupational Therapy*, 58, 446–454.

Laliberte-Rudman, D., Yu, B., Scott, E. & Pajouhandeh, P. (2000) Exploration of the perspectives of persons with schizophrenia regarding quality of life. *American Journal of Occupational Therapy*, 54 (2), 137–147.

Letts, L. (2003) Occupational therapy and participatory research: a partnership worth pursuing. *American Journal of Occupational Therapy*, 57, 77–87.

McCuaig, M. & Frank, G. (1991) The able self: adaptive patterns and choices in independent living for a person with cerebral palsy. *American Journal of Occupational Therapy*, 45, 224–234.

Mercer, G. (2002) Emancipatory disability research. In: C. Barnes, M. Oliver & L. Barton (eds), *Disability Studies Today* (pp. 228–249). Oxford, Polity.

Morse, J.M. & Richards, L. (2002) *Read Me First for a User's Guide to Qualitative Methods.* Thousand Oaks, Calif., Sage.

Mortenson, W.B. & Dyck, I. (2006) Power and client-centered practice: an insider exploration of occupational therapists' experiences. *Canadian Journal of Occupational Therapy,* 73 (5), 261–271.

Murray, R. (2004) *Writing for Academic Journals.* London, Open University Press.

Padilla, R. (2003) Clara: a phenomenology of disability. *American Journal of Occupational Therapy,* 57, 413–423.

Primeau, L.A. (2003) Reflections on self in qualitative research: stories of family. *American Journal of Occupational Therapy,* 57 (1), 9–16.

Rebeiro, K. (2004) How qualitative research evidence can inform and challenge occupational therapy practice. In: K.W. Hammell & C. Carpenter (eds), *Qualitative Research in Evidence-based Rehabilitation* (pp. 89–102). Edinburgh, Churchill Livingstone.

Rebeiro, K. & Cook, J.V. (1999) Opportunity, not prescription: an exploratory study of the experience of occupational engagement. *Canadian Journal of Occupational Therapy,* 66 (4), 176–187.

Rebeiro, K., Day, D.G., Semeniuk, B. *et al.* (2001) Northern Initiative for Social Action: an occupation-based mental health program. *American Journal of Occupational Therapy,* 55, 493–500.

Sandelowski, M. (2004) Using qualitative research. *Qualitative Health Research,* 14 (10), 1366–1386.

Schachter, C.L., Teram, E. & Stalker, C.A. (2004) Integrating grounded theory and action research to develop guidelines for sensitive practice with survivors of childhood sexual abuse. In: K.W. Hammell & C. Carpenter (eds), *Qualitative Research in Evidence-based Rehabilitation* (pp. 77–88). Edinburgh, Churchill Livingstone.

Silverman, D. (2000) *Doing Qualitative Research: a Practical Handbook.* London, Sage.

Smaling, A. (2003) Inductive, analogical, and communicative generalization. *International Journal of Qualitative Methods,* 2 (1). Article 5. Retrieved 31 March 2007 from: http://www.ualberta.ca/~iiqm/backissues/2_1/html/smaling.html

Suto, M. (2000) Issues related to data collection. In: K.W. Hammell, C. Carpenter & I. Dyck (eds), *Using Qualitative Research: a Practical Introduction for Occupational and Physical Therapists* (pp. 35–46). Edinburgh, Churchill Livingstone.

Suto, M. (2004) Exploring leisure meanings that inform client-centered practice. In: K.W. Hammell & C. Carpenter (eds), *Qualitative Research in Evidence-based Rehabilitation* (pp. 27–39). Edinburgh, Churchill Livingstone.

Teram, E., Schachter, C.L. & Stalker, C.A. (2005) The case for integrating grounded theory and participatory action research: empowering clients to inform professional practice. *Qualitative Health Research,* 15 (8), 1129–1140.

Unhuh, A.M. (2007) Reflections on . . . writing for successful publication. *Canadian Journal of Occupational Therapy,* 74 (1), 61–68.

Chapter 9

ENSURING THE QUALITY OF QUALITATIVE RESEARCH

Introduction

The proliferation of qualitative research in the rehabilitation sciences in the past two decades has advanced the theory and practice of occupational therapy and physical therapy, and perhaps more importantly, our collective understanding of the experience of chronic conditions and disability in the short and long term. This emergence of qualitative health research has made qualitative findings difficult to dismiss and has generated considerable debate about the nature of evidence-based practice. This debate is reflected in the literature of all health disciplines where 'the error of excluding qualitative research from systematic reviews of research and in adhering to biased evidence hierarchies and quality criteria that automatically exclude qualitative studies from any consideration at all, let alone consideration as best evidence' (Sandelowski, 2004, p. 1370) is being clearly articulated. The current interest in fully incorporating qualitative approaches into the research agenda upon which evidence-based practice is founded raises three important questions. First, how can the quality of qualitative research be evaluated? Second, can the level of evidence of qualitative research be evaluated? Third, how can qualitative research findings be utilized? In Chapter 8, we discussed the practical issues of disseminating qualitative research. This chapter follows on from that topic by making the argument that for qualitative research evidence to be of practical use in rehabilitation we need to be able to judge the rigor and quality of the research being conducted and to appraise the qualitative literature critically. We primarily focus in this chapter on identifying and discussing the evaluative criteria and strategies commonly used to demonstrate and appraise the rigor of qualitative research. In addition, we briefly explore issues related to classifying qualitative evidence and the utilization and translation of the knowledge generated through qualitative research.

The development of evaluative criteria for qualitative research

It is generally accepted that 'without rigor, research is worthless, becomes fiction, and loses its utility' (Morse *et al.*, 2002, p. 2). Since the imperative of evidence-based practice was established in the 1990s, much attention has focused on establishing the reliability and validity of research. Initially, the quality or 'validity' of qualitative inquiry was judged by applying the reliability and validity standards of quantitative or experimental research based on a positivist philosophy. These traditional standards, broadly defined, were considered applicable and appropriate benchmarks by which qualitative research could be judged. Reliability referred to the stability of findings, whereas validity represented the truthfulness of findings (Altheide & Johnson, 1994). Concerns were raised, however, about the incompatibility of these terms with the ontological, epistemological and methodological foundations of qualitative inquiry, but the need remained to convince 'the dominant and somewhat hostile scientific community about the merits of qualitative research' (Whittemore *et al.*, 2001, p. 523). The philosophical differences between qualitative and quantitative inquiry have been clearly delineated (for example Smith, 1993) and greatly influenced the evolution of translated evaluative criteria for qualitative research. A lively debate about qualitative research criteria continues, with some authors making 'a plea for the return to terminology for ensuring rigor that is used by mainstream science' (Morse *et al.*, 2002, p. 1). Until the last decade, occupational therapy and physical therapy education programs focused primarily on the skills needed to conduct and critically appraise quantitative (and less so survey) methodologies. In our experience, even though these programs have been expanded to include qualitative methodologies, students still find it difficult to reconceptualize and apply the traditional standards of reliability and validity beyond the rationale established for quantitative inquiry. For this reason, as teachers and researchers in physical therapy and occupational therapy, we prefer to introduce students and practitioners to the translated evaluative criteria terms developed specifically for qualitative inquiry.

In developing criteria for qualitative research, scholars have to take into consideration the contextual, subjective and interpretive nature of qualitative inquiry, different methodological perspectives and the integral role of the researcher. Qualitative research findings can be interesting, evocative, illuminating and yet erroneous (Miles & Huberman, 1994). The use of "erroneous" in this context does not refer to a right or wrong judgment about the results of research, but rather to interpretive qualitative findings that cannot be substantiated or are reflective only of researcher "bias" and agenda. There appears to be consensus among scholars that 'some kind of validity criteria and some methodological or technical procedures [what we later call strategies] are essential to guard against the investigator's conjuring up concepts and theories that do not authentically represent the phenomenon of concern' (Whittemore *et al.*, 2001, p. 526). Numerous scholars have contributed to developing common validity criteria in qualitative research but Lincoln & Guba's (1985) contribution has been particularly influential. The translated evaluative criteria they developed remain the "gold standard" and it is these that we will discuss more comprehensively in this chapter.

Evaluating qualitative research

'Evaluative criteria are the basic principles used to guide the judgment of the integrity or trustworthiness of a study' (Baxter & Eyles, 1997, p. 506). According to Smith & Deemer (2000), 'criteria should not be thought of in abstraction but as a list of features that we think, or more or less agree at any given time and place, characterize good versus bad inquiry' (p. 894). Their comment highlights the dynamic nature of qualitative criteria that are always being challenged and debated, applied in practice and modified. Those who adopt a relativist stance 'also recognize the need for and value of plurality, multiplicity, the acceptance and celebration of differences' (Smith & Deemer, 2000, p. 894). Evaluative criteria that are described like this seem unsatisfactory and confusing to those who are used to the certainty associated with quantitative research. However, it is an ethical obligation for researchers to ensure the rigor and integrity of their research by appropriately articulating which evaluative criteria they used and how they addressed them in designing the study.

Lincoln & Guba (1985) proposed four criteria as a translation of the more traditional terms associated with quantitative research: internal validity to *credibility*, external validity to *transferability*, reliability to *dependability* and objectivity to *confirmability* (see Table 9.1). The criterion of transferability has alternatively been described as *applicability* (Guba & Lincoln, 1989) and confirmability as *trustworthiness* (Eisner, 1991) or *authenticity* (Sandelowski, 1986) and the terms are frequently used interchangeably.

Credibility and authenticity are concerned with determining whether the research is genuine, reliable, or authoritative, that is, whether the findings can be trusted. It refers to the researcher's meticulous efforts to establish confidence in the integrity of the data analysis and interpretive findings. Credibility is based on the constructivist assumption that there is no single reality but rather multiple realities that are constructed by people in their own contexts and require authentic representations of experience that can be seen as plausible by the participants.

Transferability or applicability asks the question: 'To what degree can the study findings be generalized or applied to other individuals or groups, contexts or settings?' It refers to the degree to which qualitative findings inform and facilitate

Table 9.1 Evaluative criteria in qualitative and quantitative research.

Qualitative research	Quantitative research	
Credibility	Internal validity	Generalizability
Transferablility	External validity	
Dependability	Reliability	
Confirmability	Objectivity	

insights within contexts other than that in which the research was conducted. This important criterion is discussed in more depth later in this chapter.

Dependability is concerned with how the findings of the study – whether in the form of description, interpretation, or theory – 'fit' the data from which they have been derived. It refers to the plausibility of the design decisions taken and implemented by the researcher. This criterion has been associated with the terms 'decision' or 'audit trail', by which researchers account for their methodological choices and data collection methods, and develop coherent linkages between the data and reported findings. This audit trail enables the reader to judge the adequacy of the research process.

Lincoln & Guba (1985) describe confirmability as 'the degree to which findings are determined by the respondents and conditions of the inquiry and not by the biases, motivations, interests or perspectives of the inquirer' (p. 290). This criterion focuses primarily on the role of the researcher within the research process and how their location, values, beliefs, ideologies and theoretical stance influence the data analysis process and the findings.

The validity or evaluative criteria we have described are not rigid rules but rather they serve as guiding principles or anchor points for determining the integrity and evaluating the relevance and utility of qualitative research. They do not, however, ensure that the research *will be* relevant and useful. A number of common techniques or strategies have been identified which can be employed to demonstrate or assure specific validity criteria (Whittemore *et al.*, 2001). These strategies of rigor do not in themselves *ensure* the trustworthiness of the research. They need to be selectively employed, adapted and combined to achieve the purposes of specific studies, and their use is justified by linking strategy decisions with the research question and design.

Strategies used for ensuring rigor

Verification of research is 'the process of checking, confirming, making sure, and being certain' (Morse *et al.*, 2002, p. 9) and is achieved by the researcher's creative, sensitive, flexible and critical use of selected strategies. These strategies help the researcher identify when to continue, stop or modify the research process and are woven into every step of the research planning and implementation process (Morse *et al.*, 2002). A summary of the most commonly described strategies associated with elements of the research process is provided in Table 9.2.

Rationale for methodological decisions

In Chapter 4, we discussed a number of methodologies (grounded theory, phenomenology, ethnography and participatory action research) that inform and guide the design of qualitative studies. Methodological justification contributes to the integrity of research design decisions and forges links between the research aim, choice of methods and data analysis approach. It is not, however, sufficient to simply state that 'this study used grounded theory to generate its findings' or 'this

Table 9.2 Strategies for demonstrating rigor.

Research process	Strategies of rigor
Study design	Rationale provided for methodological decisions Establishing an audit or decision trail
Data collection or generation	Appropriate sampling strategies Data saturation Triangulation
Data analysis process	Member checking Peer review In-depth rich description
Presentation of findings	Reflexivity Representation Providing evidence to support interpretations

study employed phenomenological methods' (Avis, 2003, p. 1003). Researchers need to be explicit about their research decisions and processes, to provide what Thorne (1997) describes as 'the detailed design-logic descriptions that convince audiences that researchers are aware of the implications of the chosen method-ological foundation' (p. 292).

Some health care research represents what could be described as a 'blurred genre' (Denzin & Lincoln, 2005, p. 3) approach. These primarily descriptive or exploratory studies are usually small in scale and are described in terms of their focus on one data collection method, usually interviews or focus groups. We acknowledge that for these researchers it may be difficult to ground their research in a particular methodology. However, we consider it important that they make their ontolo-gical and epistemological positions clear by selecting the key philosophical sys-tem (interpretivism, constructivism and critical theory), discussed in Chapter 2, that informs their purpose and approach. The qualitative research process is rarely linear and as it progresses the research purpose or question may shift, sampling strategies may be changed and data generation methods modified. The flexible nature of qualitative research requires that these components fit with the analysis pro-cess, that each remains congruent with the previous component and the guiding methodological assumptions to form a coherent whole (Morse *et al.*, 2002). A full explanation of these decisions is essential to ensure methodological and the-oretical congruence.

Establishing an audit or decision trail

The idea of an audit trail is analogous to a fiscal audit in that someone external to the research process checks on the status of the research to ensure that appro-priate decisions are being made along the way (Baxter & Eyles, 1997). The term is used synonymously with 'decision trail' and is intended to produce a detailed account of how the research was conducted and includes tracking the decisions made in recruiting participants, collecting data and the analytic approach taken in transforming the data into findings. The latter is particularly important as the audit trail provides evidence that the findings are representative of the data set as a whole. The purpose is to provide readers with the comprehensive information they need to verify the dependability of the research. However, as Letts *et al.* (2007) point out, 'researchers often confront space limitations in publishing their research, so frequently state that they have used a decision trail, but may not provide all the details' (p. 9).

Sampling decisions and data saturation

Purposive sampling strategies are primarily used in qualitative research and in Chapter 5 we described a number of purposive sampling approaches based on the specific purpose or aim of the research. The aim of sampling in qualitative research is to select an appropriate sample. This consists of participants who best represent and have specific knowledge, experience or expertise of the research topic. The sampling process is flexible and at the beginning of the study the number of participants to be involved is usually uncertain. The main indicators of sample adequacy in qualitative research are redundancy, data or theoretical saturation and replication. Sample adequacy ensures that the emerging themes have been efficiently and effectively saturated with optimal quality data and that 'sufficient data to account for all aspects of the phenomenon have been obtained' (Morse *et al.*, 2002, p. 12). It is important to differentiate the notion of 'saturating' participants from data saturation. As Morse *et al.* (2002) warn, 'one of the most common mistakes is that new investigators repeatedly interview the same participants until nothing new emerges' (p. 16), rather than saturating the data by purposively recruiting more new participants until the data set is as complete as possible. Researchers also need to be aware that some sampling strategies, for example snowball sampling, can lead to self-selection 'biases' which can influence the sample characteristics. The 'skewed' sample may be purposeful and adventageous, but the influence on the data acquired needs to be acknowledged and reported by the researcher.

Triangulation

The concept of triangulation 'arises by means of analogy with a process adopted in navigation, whereby the position of an object can be more accurately determined by taking two or more bearings upon it' (Sim & Sharp, 1998, p. 23). Triangulation is viewed as one of the most powerful strategies for strengthening credibility and is based on the convergence of information from multiple sources to corroborate the data and evolving themes. The combination of multiple sources adds rigor, breadth, complexity, richness and depth to an inquiry (Denzin & Lincoln, 2005).

Three types of triangulation are commonly used in health care research and involve the use of multiple methods, data or sources and researchers. Method triangulation is basically the use of more than one method of data collection in a study;

for example Eysenbach & Kohler (2002) used focus groups, participant observation and in-depth interviews in their study of how consumers search for and appraise health information on the World Wide Web. Source or data triangulation usually refers to the involvement of multiple participants or the use of multiple data quotes to corroborate, elaborate or illuminate an emerging theme or the phenomenon of interest. It might also be achieved by expanding the locations or sites where data are being collected; for example when conducting an institutional ethnography, occupational therapists could be observed in a diversity of settings, such as different inpatient wards and outpatient departments within one hospital. However, simply using more than one method or source does not necessarily guarantee findings that are more rigorous. Furthermore, Baxter & Eyles (1997) observe that few researchers comment on their rationale for using several methods, explain whether they think these address the same or different questions, or explore the discrepancies in the data generated from multiple sources. Researcher triangulation usually occurs when researchers work as a team investigating the same or a similar topic; for example Thorne *et al.* (2004) formed a multidisciplinary team interested in understanding health care communication issues from the perspective of people with multiple sclerosis. Based on their interpretive findings, the authors recommended a number of communication competencies for those who provide nursing and rehabilitation services for people with this chronic condition. Involvement of a number of researchers, each contributing to data collection and analysis, can be seen as an advantage as their different perspectives can enrich the research process.

Member checking

Member checking, also called member validation, is a process whereby the researcher seeks clarification and further explanation from the participants involved in the study. The strategy appeals because it reflects some core values of qualitative research related to accurate representation, privileging participants' knowledge and experience, and decreasing the power imbalances between researcher and participant. There is an ethical imperative to inform the participants about the research findings and about how the findings are being used (Miles & Huberman, 1994). Baxter & Eyles (1997) suggest that 'member checking should be done in the spirit of an exchange of ideas' (p. 515). There is no definitive procedure for member checking and it can occur at virtually any stage of the research process. Participants are commonly asked, early in the research process, to review their interview or focus group transcript and add or delete information they regret saying or, alternatively, think would make an additional contribution. During the analysis stage, participants can be asked to review the data in abstracted form (categories or preliminary themes), or as an executive summary or draft chapter. Essentially, their involvement at these stages is to validate the researcher's interpretive process, to determine whether the participants are able to 'hear their own voices', or have their experiences or perspectives represented, in the preliminary findings.

Involvement of participants at these higher levels of data analysis does present some difficulties. Without being involved in the particulars of the analytic process, participants may feel ill-equipped to comment beyond their own data, perceive the findings as too abstract to relate to their own experience, or reject the interpretation as not being congruent with their values or self-image (Miles & Huberman, 1994). When evaluating the usefulness of member checking for a specific study it is important to consider how the strategy might affect the participant and what to do if the participant has widely differing opinions on the emerging findings. Carpenter (2004) explored dilemmas of practice as experienced by physical therapists in rehabilitation settings and provides an example of how member checking can be integrated effectively into the data analysis phase. During the data reduction phase of the analysis stage, she wrote a detailed description of each of six preliminary themes that she perceived to be emerging from the data. Five participants had expressed an interest in reviewing these theme descriptions during the data collection phase. Carpenter sent this material to them with a letter explaining that this was one stage in the data analysis process and asking them to consider the following questions in their deliberations:

- In what ways do these themes capture (or not) your own experiences of dilemmas as described during the interviews or currently?
- Is there a way, based on your experience, that you could more precisely state these dilemma themes?
- Is there anything you would add to these theme descriptions that would make them more relevant to your experience?

Each of the five participants returned the descriptions with detailed written comments and suggestions and these were incorporated into the next phase of data analysis. Involving all or some of the participants in a review of the research materials ensures that the researcher has accurately translated their perspectives, decreases the chances of misrepresentation or appropriation, and strengthens the linkages between interpretation and the original data (Carpenter & Hammell, 2000).

Peer review

This strategy is also called peer or expert checking and involves a peer who is a colleague not involved with the study but who has a general understanding of the study topic and of qualitative research approaches. This person is asked to review field notes and transcripts analytically in order to validate or question the linkages being established between the data, categories and codes, and emerging themes. As Lincoln & Guba (1985) suggest, peer review is one way of keeping the researcher honest, and the searching questions that result from this process may contribute to a deeper reflexive analysis. In a study exploring the experience of spinal cord injury from the individual perspective, Carpenter (2000) asked a colleague, who possessed knowledge of spinal cord injury and qualitative research, to identify units of meaning from intact transcript copies and to assign them to the categories using the definitions that had been developed. Discrepancies that arose between their respective decisions caused Carpenter to reflect and to define the categories more clearly before reducing them further to themes. However, as Carpenter & Hammell (2000) warn, 'it is important to emphasize that peer review is designed to help clarify the researcher's perspectives; the peer does not represent a standard against which the findings are compared; nor is it an attempt to obtain a second opinion' (p. 111). There are also real dangers 'that one person may defer to the other on the basis of unequal power/relations' (Baxter & Eyles, 1997, p. 514), particularly if the researcher is a graduate student or novice researcher and the peer reviewer is the supervisor or a more experienced researcher.

In-depth and rich description

Writing is an important skill for qualitative researchers to develop. The reader of qualitative research should be provided with an in-depth and 'thick description' (Geertz, 1973) of all the important aspects of the research design, particularly those associated with the generation of data, that is, the participants, the participant–researcher relationship and the research context. A detailed profile of the participants should be provided without contravening the ethical issues of confidentiality and anonymity. In qualitative research, the participants are chosen for their unique characteristics and knowledge and, as such, when carefully selected they lend credibility to the study. Qualitative research is concerned with the context in which the topic of interest is experienced. Information about the context helps to ground and contribute to the transferability of the findings. Field notes, reflective journals and analytic memos all contribute, if diligently maintained by the researcher throughout the process, to this 'thick description'. Prolonged engagement, a concept derived from ethnography, involves spending sufficient time in the field to build trust and rapport between the researcher and participants and to gain an in-depth knowledge of the study context. The concept is usually associated with participant observation, but may take the form of a number of interviews with each participant over time or immersion in reviewing and analyzing documents or records. Morse *et al.* (2002) also recommend keeping a meticulous record of the theory development process that they describe as moving 'with deliberation between a micro perspective of the data and macro conceptual/theoretical understanding' (p. 13). 'Thick description' does not just entail an extensive description of all relevant aspects of the study. It includes a description of the several meanings that are possible within the study context, what Geertz (1973) describes as 'a stratified hierarchy of meaning structures' (p. 7). The researcher cannot describe everything in detail, especially when faced with the word limits imposed by peer-reviewed journals, and so has to make decisions about what information to prioritize and consider how the findings might be applied and inform other situations.

Reflexivity

Reflexivity is an essential strategy that is integral to the whole research process, not just as a means of verifying the credibility or authenticity of the research. The concept of reflexivity recognizes that the researcher is an integral part of the research process and demands a full assessment of the influence of the researcher's background, perceptions and interests on the research design and findings. The issues of reflexivity have been touched on throughout this book and discussed in detail in Chapter 7. It is central to establishing the integrity and critical abilities of the researcher and 'must be evidenced in the process to assure that the interpretation is valid and grounded within the data' (Whittemore *et al.*, 2001, p. 531). The researcher must be critical and diligent in searching for alternative interpretations and rival explanations, in exploring negative cases or instances and examining personal 'biases' (Miles & Huberman, 1994). As Miles & Huberman (1994) state, 'a good look at the [often inconvenient] exceptions can test and strengthen the findings – tests the generality and protects [the researcher] against self-selecting biases and helps build a better explanation' (p. 269). Negative case or instance analysis involves an inductive process of revising an interpretation by comparing it with all the data until it accounts for all known cases (Baxter & Eyles, 1997). It encourages the researcher to explore all dimensions of the emerging themes in order to ensure a robust analytic process and is particularly recommended in grounded theory where the aim is development of a theory. Reflexivity is a complex strategy that is characteristic of qualitative research and underpins the integrity and critical nature of the knowledge claims made by researchers.

Providing evidence to support interpretations

Participant verbatim quotations frequently represent the primary data of qualitative research and, as such, are important 'for revealing how meanings are expressed in the respondents' own words rather the words of the researcher' (Baxter & Eyles, 1997, p. 508). The use of quotations in reporting study findings varies greatly. Some researchers provide many quotes with little accompanying commentary, while others provide few quotes with considerable commentary (Carpenter & Hammell, 2000). Under these circumstances, the reader is required to judge whether the verbatim quotations provided inform and support the researchers' interpretations and represent the thematic findings. In addition, 'the selection of some words and not others, the voices of some participants and not others represents the power of researchers [within] the research process and the choices made based on their understandings and agendas' (Carpenter & Hammell, 2000, p. 114). These choices must, therefore, be explained and justified. In general, the inclusion of selected quotations is considered important in presenting qualitative findings. Increasingly, peer-reviewed journals acknowledge the need to assign an increased word limit to qualitative studies to accommodate for this inclusion of pertinent data.

Generalizability or transferability of qualitative findings

The criteria of credibility and transferability have been linked in efforts to provide a rationale for the 'generalizability' of qualitative research. The generalizability of research findings has been considered the prerogative of quantitative research

(Morse, 1999) and not the purpose of qualitative research (Sandelowski, 1986). Generalizability in quantitative research is achieved by ensuring external validity through such strategies as an adequate random sample and comparison of that sample with the larger population. 'Using this standard, qualitative research, with small and purposefully selected samples, has been considered non-representative of the population and therefore not generalizable' (Morse, 1999, p. 5). The criterion of transferability focuses on the theoretical or analytical generalizability of qualitative findings. The theoretical knowledge gained from qualitative research is applicable beyond the immediate group to all similar situations, questions and individuals or groups (Morse, 1999; Sandelowski, 2004).

Of course, as Smaling (2003) suggests, 'every research project need not lead to results and conclusions that are generalizable [or transferable]' (p. 2). For example, the findings of a study designed to evaluate a particular program in a specific, unique setting need not be transferable to other organizations or programs. Transferability is implicitly based on analogical reasoning (Smaling, 2003). Readers of a research report, rather than the researcher, determine whether analogies exist between the situation that has been researched and another situation that is of interest to them. The researcher's responsibility is to provide sufficient detailed information about the study design and implementation (thick description and an audit trail) to enable the reader to make a judgment about the quality and rigor of the study and the applicability of the findings to their specific practical experience. More recently, this tendency to shift responsibility for transferability to the readers of research reports has been challenged in relation to research utilization and knowledge translation (Sandelowski, 2004). Researchers are now expected to improve the 'utilization value' of their reports (Smaling, 2003, p. 20) by discussing the levels and applications of qualitative evidence and writing for different user groups, including client groups who might benefit as well as practitioners and policy makers.

Critical appraisal of qualitative research

The broad term 'qualitative research' encapsulates a variety of methodological approaches and methods. The flexibility of qualitative approaches and the capacity to adapt to different research settings is seen as an inherent strength (Daly *et al.*, 2007). This same flexibility is not so easily captured in the definitive evaluative criteria approaches developed for experimental research, for example the checklist developed for the Physiotherapy Evidence Database (PEDro) (2007). This checklist consists of ten scale items addressing such criteria as random allocation, comparability of groups at baseline and analysis by intention to treat. Decisions about the validity of clinical trials are rated according to an overall score out of ten. Such scoring systems can be used to determine the strength or level of quantitative research evidence and whether a study should be included in a systematic review. Qualitative researchers have resisted a checklist approach, arguing that it would fail to capture the nuances and intricacies of qualitative research and constrain the flexibility and creativity characteristic of these approaches. While experienced qualitative researchers can undoubtedly critically appraise the quality and rigor of qualitative studies, the lack of explicit guidelines for evaluating qualitative studies has made it difficult for those investigators newly exploring qualitative research. Recently, there has been considerable interest in developing explicit guidelines for assessing qualitative research, for example the Cochrane Qualitative Methods Group (2002). A number of critical appraisal frameworks have been developed, for example Letts *et al.* (2007) and the British Sociological Association (1996), that are compatible with the underlying theoretical assumptions of the various qualitative methodologies. However, there is currently no consensus on what would constitute a satisfactory appraisal tool for qualitative research for use within the Cochrane Collaboration. An evaluative framework, based on a summary of the criteria and strategies to enhance rigor discussed in this chapter (see Table 9.3), provides suggestions for critically appraising qualitative research papers.

Establishing the quality and rigor of research is fundamental to evidence-based practice. The definition of 'best' evidence has been primarily associated with 'scientific' evidence derived from experimental research. The development of clearly defined criteria and hierarchies or levels of quantitative evidence, where evidence from at least one systematic review (with homogeneity) of multiple randomized controlled trials is considered Level 1 (Sackett *et al.*, 2000), has facilitated the determination of 'best' evidence. Critics have suggested that traditional reliance upon quantitative evidence by rehabilitation professionals has contributed to the apparent theory–practice gap, wherein the research undertaken had little or no relevance to the realities of clinical practice.

In response, there is an increasing desire to utilize evidence from qualitative research, but this has proved difficult for a number of reasons. The need to develop a recognized approach to critical appraisal of qualitative research is currently being addressed but, as Sandelowski & Barroso (2003) suggest, finding the findings in qualitative research can be a problem. There is much greater variation in the style of reporting qualitative research than in quantitative research reports 'where a harder line is typically drawn between results and discussion' (Sandelowski & Barroso, 2003, p. 905). The utility of conducting qualitative research meta-syntheses (or systematic reviews) is recognized (discussed in Chapter 10), but the issue of classifying and integrating the findings presents a problem. Sandelowski & Barroso (2003) define qualitative findings as 'the data-driven and integrated discoveries, judgment, and/or pronouncements researchers offer about the phenomenon, events, or cases under investigation' (p. 909). This broader, more abstract definition of findings is in contrast to the generally statistical nature of quantitative results, which are more conducive to checklists and rating scales.

Despite these difficulties, there is considerable interest in developing classifications, typologies or hierarchies of qualitative findings. Kearney (2001) proposed 'five categories of qualitative findings: those restricted by a priori frameworks, descriptive categories, shared pathway or meaning, depiction of experiential variation, and dense explanatory description' (p. 145); and several ways by which qualitative evidence could be applied to clinical practice. She bases her levels of qualitative

Table 9.3 Qualitative research critical appraisal framework.

Critical appraisal of qualitative research article	
Components of article	**Questions to ask in article review**
Study purpose	• Is the purpose/objective/aim clearly articulated? • Is it referred to consistently throughout the article?
Literature review	• Is sufficient background for the study provided? • Are terms/concepts defined as used in the study? • Do the authors use relevant literature to adequately justify the need for the study? • Is the literature current and related to the purpose of the study? • If appropriate, do the references reflect current professional knowledge?
Study design	• Do the authors describe their methodological approach? • Is a coherent argument made for its appropriateness for the study purpose? • Is the researcher's theoretical perspective or conceptual framework articulated?
Research methods	• Are the methods used to recruit participants and collect data thoroughly described and justified? • Are the ethical issues addressed (including informed consent, relationship of researcher to the participant, ethical review, permission obtained to audiotape/video/observe)?
Location of researcher	• Are issues of positionality (initial interest in topic, background and experience as it impacts the research) and reflexivity (how do researcher values, beliefs and assumptions influence the research process) addressed?
Data analysis process	• Is the analysis process adequately described? • Are the findings clearly and fully documented? • Are data (participant quotes) used to substantiate the findings? • Is the researcher's decision trail clearly described? • Has a rationale for the interpretation of the findings been provided?
Strategies used to enhance rigor	• Were strategies (for example triangulation, or peer and member checking) appropriately selected and incorporated into the study design and fully described?
Discussion of findings	• Does the discussion relate to the stated purpose of the research? • Are the findings related to the literature review? • Is new literature introduced to support the study findings or implications? • Are tensions and similarities between the study findings and other research identified? • Is the language used appropriate for the research approach and the participants' role in the process?
Conclusions	• Are the implications for clinical practice and future research discussed? • Is the transferability (generalizability) of the research discussed? • Have the limitations of the research study been identified?

evidence not only on the fit of the research findings with clinical issues but 'also on the richness and informativeness of the findings as evidence' (p. 146). Richness of the findings can be characterized as a combination of complexity and discovery. Complexity relates to the interweaving of components of the findings with the participants' particular experiences and circumstances, contextual details and political influences. Discovery is defined as 'the presentation by researchers of new perspectives on, or information about, the human phenomenon under study' (Kearney, 2001, p. 146).

Sandelowski & Barroso (2003) independently developed a typology of qualitative findings that nevertheless bears a striking similarity to Kearney's (2001) levels of evidence. Their typology consists of five components and places 'qualitative findings on a continuum indicating transformation of data' (p. 908). The first two components of the continuum were not recognized as qualitative research. 'No-findings reports' present the data as if they were findings, without any effort to describe or interpret more abstractly, and topical surveys were characterized by nominal or categorical data, or lists and inventories of topics covered by research participants in interviews and focus groups. Thematic survey, the third component, represents an exploratory approach and offers a 'more penetrating or nuanced description of experience, using the everyday language of the participants or themes or concepts from existing empirical or theoretical literature to organize the data' (Sandelowski & Barroso, 2003, p. 912). Conceptual or thematic description is described as the fourth component of the typology. This descriptive approach is characterized by a more complex and systematic approach to data analysis in which the data is abstracted and organized according to underlying patterns and presented as a number of themes or concepts. Interpretive explanation represents the most complex component of the continuum and offers a coherent dense explanatory model or the essence of a phenomenon. These authors focused on the quality and utility of the findings to practice rather than the methodological type and rigor. They emphasize differences between qualitative findings not differences in quality between qualitative studies. In our opinion, such approaches to classifying qualitative evidence can assist healthcare practitioners and researchers to identify the type of knowledge generated and the support it provides for 'best' practice and to integrate the findings of qualitative studies in meta-syntheses.

Other authors (Cesario et al., 2002; Daly et al., 2007) have focused on developing a numeric scoring system based on an evaluative framework or a hierarchy according to methodological type. These approaches reflect the more traditional approaches to assessing research evidence originally developed for quantitative research. Cesario et al. (2002) developed a scoring system of zero to three that could be applied to five categories of qualitative evaluative criteria and used to rate the quality of qualitative studies. The designation of a high score indicates a high-level, well-constructed, qualitative study. Daly et al. (2007) propose a hierarchy of evidence consisting of four levels. According to this hierarchy, the least likely studies (Level 1) to produce good evidence-for-practice are single case studies, followed by descriptive studies that may provide helpful lists of quotations but do not offer detailed analysis.

More weight is given to conceptual studies that analyze all data according to conceptual themes but may be limited by a lack of diversity of sample. Generalizable studies using conceptual frameworks to derive an appropriately diversified sample with analysis accounting for all the data are considered to provide the best evidence-for-practice (Daly *et al.*, 2007, p. 43).

Development of such hierarchies is complicated by the multiple methodological and method combinations that characterize qualitative research, and in fact, the hierarchy described here was confined to studies using interviews as the method of data collection.

Issues of knowledge translation

It is clear to us that it is important for health qualitative researchers to fully engage in the discussions about how to appraise qualitative studies critically, and classify and integrate qualitative evidence. There are risks in attempting to reduce the complexities and nuances of qualitative research to a simple criteria checklist or numeric score and this endeavor may in fact not be desirable. However, practitioners unfamiliar with the intricacies of qualitative methodologies do benefit from evaluative guidelines in developing their appraisal skills. In addition, understanding and evaluating claims to knowledge made by qualitative research is important in meeting policy and practice demands of an increasingly complex health care environment. These issues underpin the concept of knowledge translation or transfer. The Canadian Institutes of Health Research (2004) define knowledge translation as:

> The exchange, synthesis, and ethically-sound application of knowledge – within a complex set of interactions among researchers and users – to accelerate the capture of the benefits of research for Canadians through improved health, more effective services and products, and a strengthened health care system.

Knowledge translation is a relatively new concept that is used to describe a relatively old problem – the underutilization of research evidence in systems of care, such as rehabilitation services (Davis *et al.*, 2003). The term may appear similar to dissemination but 'it can be differentiated by its emphasis on the quality of research prior to dissemination and implementation of research evidence within a system' (National Center for the Dissemination of Disability Research, 2005, p. 1). Researchers have long accepted the responsibility to disseminate their research findings, but the concept of 'knowledge translation involves more than distribution of practical scientific information and reliance on academic publication as a primary mechanism for disseminating results' (National Center for the Dissemination of Disability Research, NCDDR, 2005, p. 1).

In Canada and the UK, where the term is commonly used, researchers have focused on knowledge translation (or transfer) as both a process and a strategy that can lead to the utilization of research findings by individual practitioners, organizations and governments and improved outcomes for consumers, students and patients

(NCDDR, 2005). Researchers are now expected 'to develop the clinical acumen to move research findings into practice' (Sandelowski & Barroso, 2003, p. 1381) and to identify how their research findings can contribute to knowledge translation. These expectations are reflected in a number of strategies adopted by peer-reviewed journals, for example clinical commentaries on specific research papers. Numerous knowledge translation planning models or frameworks have been developed, consisting of multiple stages to assist researchers and health care planners to identify research gaps and plan for evidence-based implementation. Jacobsen *et al.* (2003) offer one such framework for audience-centered knowledge translation that comprises five key domains: user group, issue, research, research–user relationship and dissemination strategy. The NCDDR (2005), however, suggests that many of these frameworks need to be refined to 'reflect the context in which end-users of high-quality information will make decisions, solve problems, or use knowledge as consumers, practitioners or educators in their everyday lives' (p. 4). In order to embrace this more participative view, the NCDDR (2005) have recommended that the following new definition of knowledge translation be adopted:

> The collaborative and systematic review, assessment, identification, aggregation, and practical application of high-quality disability and rehabilitation research by key stakeholders (i.e. consumers, researchers, practitioners, and policy makers) for improving the lives of individuals with disabilities (p. 4).

Qualitative researchers must assume and share responsibility for translating the findings of their research. This means conducting ethical and rigorous studies, clarifying what constitutes qualitative evidence, and integrating qualitative findings in meaningful ways. Sandelowski & Barroso (2003) suggest that the distinction between *users* of knowledge and *producers* of knowledge is an artificial one. As they point out:

> Researchers use the findings of other researchers . . . to produce their own findings, which are then used to generate other studies, the findings of which will be disseminated for use by others. Research findings are used whenever anyone disseminates, translates, implements and evaluates them (p. 1380).

We concur with Sandelowski & Barroso's (2003) opinion that 'qualitative health research is the best thing to be happening to evidence-based practice' (p. 1382), but we are aware that the imperative of evidence-based practice directs us, as researchers, to take seriously the issues of qualitative research and knowledge translation. In the last chapter, we will discuss other important developments in qualitative research related to the participant–researcher relationship, the increasing use of mixed methods research approaches, meta-synthesis of qualitative findings and use of the Internet and email by qualitative researchers.

References

Altheide, D.L. & Johnson, J.M. (1994) Criteria for assessing interpretive validity in qualitative research. In: N.K. Denzin & Y.S. Lincoln (eds), *Handbook of Qualitative Research* (pp. 485–499). Thousand Oaks, Calif., Sage.

Avis, M. (2003) Do we need methodological theory to do qualitative research? *Qualitative Health Research*, 13 (7), 995–1004.

Baxter, J. & Eyles, J. (1997) Evaluating qualitative research in social geography: establishing 'rigour' in interview analysis. *Transactions of the Institute of British Geographers*, 22, 505–525.

British Sociological Association Medical Sociology Group (1996) *Criteria for the Evaluation of Qualitative Research Papers*. Retrieved 12 April 2007 from: http://www.tandf.co.uk/journals/pdf/qdr.pdf

Canadian Institutes of Health Research (2004) *Knowledge Translation Strategy 2004–2009: Innovation in Action*. Retrieved 2 April 2007 from: http://www.cihr~irsc.gc.ca/e/26574.html#defining

Carpenter, C. (2000) Exploring the lived experience of disability. In: K.W. Hammell, C. Carpenter & I. Dyck (eds), *Using Qualitative Research: a Practical Introduction for Occupational and Physical Therapists* (pp. 23–33). Edinburgh, Churchill Livingstone.

Carpenter, C. (2004) Dilemmas of practice as experienced by physical therapists in rehabilitation settings. *Physiotherapy Canada*, 57 (1), 63–74.

Carpenter, C. & Hammell, K.W. (2000) Evaluating qualitative research. In: K.W. Hammell, C. Carpenter & I. Dyck (eds), *Using Qualitative Research: a Practical Introduction for Occupational and Physical Therapists* (pp. 107–119). Edinburgh, Churchill Livingstone.

Cesario, S., Morin, K. & Santa-Donato, A. (2002) Evaluating the level of evidence of qualitative research. *Journal of Obstetric, Gynecologic, and Neonatal Nursing*, 31 (6), 708–714.

Cochrane Qualitative Methods Group (2002) Retrieved 12 March 2007 from: http://www.joannabriggs.edu.au/cqrmg/index.html

Daley, J., Willis, K., Small, R. *et al.* (2007) A hierarchy of evidence for assessing qualitative health research. *Journal of Clinical Epidemiology*, 60, 43–49.

Davis, D., Evans, M., Jadad, A. *et al.* (2003) The case for knowledge translation: shortening the journey from evidence to effect. *British Medical Journal*, 327 (7405), 33–35.

Denzin, N.K. & Lincoln Y.S. (2005) Introduction: the discipline and practice of qualitative research. In: N.K. Denzin & Y.S. Lincoln (eds), *The Sage Handbook of Qualitative Research*, (pp. 1–32). Thousand Oaks, Calif., Sage.

Eisner, E. (1991) *The Enlightened Eye: Qualitative Inquiry and the Enhancement of Educational Practices*. New York, MacMillan.

Eysenbach, G. & Kohler, C. (2002) How do consumers search for and appraise health information on the World Wide Web? Qualitative study using focus groups, usability tests and in-depth interviews. *British Medical Journal*, 324, 573–577.

Geertz, C. (1973) *The Interpretation of Cultures: Selected Essays*. New York, Basic Books.

Guba, E.R. & Lincoln, Y.S. (1989) *Fourth Generation Evaluation*. Newbury Park, Calif., Sage.

Jacobsen, N., Butterill, D. & Goering, P. (2003) Development of a framework for knowledge translation: understanding user context. *Journal of Health Services Research & Policy*, 8 (2), 94–99.

Kearney, M. (2001) Levels and applications of qualitative research evidence. *Research in Nursing & Health*, 24, 145–153.

Letts, L., Wilkins, S., Law, M., Stewart, D., Bosch, J. & Westmorland, M. (2007) *Guidelines for Critical Review Form: Qualitative Studies (Version 2.0)*. Hamilton, McMaster University. Retrieved 31 March 2007 from: http://www.fhs.mcmaster.ca/rehab/ebp/

Lincoln, Y.S. & Guba, E.A. (1985) *Naturalistic Inquiry*. Beverly Hills, Calif., Sage.

Miles, M.B. & Huberman, A.M. (1994) *Qualitative Data Analysis* (2nd edn). Thousand Oaks, Calif., Sage.

Morse J.M. (1999) Editorial: qualitative generalizability. *Qualitative Health Research*, 9 (1), 5–6.

Morse, J., Barrett, M., Mayan, M., Olson, K. & Spiers, J. (2002) Verification strategies for establishing reliability and validity in qualitative research. *International Journal of Qualitative Methods*, 1 (2), Article 2. Retrieved 14 September 2006 from: http//: www.ualberta.ca/~ijqm/english/engframeset.htm

National Center for the Dissemination of Disability Research (2005) *Technical Brief Number 10: What is Knowledge Translation?* Retrieved 2 April 2007 from: http:// www.ncddr.org/products/focus/focus10/Focus10.pdf

Physiotherapy Evidence Database (PEDro) (2007) *Rating Clinical Trials.* Retrieved 12 April 2007 from: http://www.pedro.fhs.usyd.edu.au/scale_item.html

Sackett, D.L., Strauss, S.E., Richardson, W.S., Rosenburg, W. & Haynes, R.B. (2000) *Evidence-based Medicine: How to Practice and Teach EBM* (2nd edn). Edinburgh, Churchill Livingstone.

Sandelowski, M. (1986) The problem of rigor in qualitative research. *Advances in Nursing Science*, 8, 27–37.

Sandelowski, M. (2004) Using qualitative research. *Qualitative Health Research*, 14 (10), 1366–1386.

Sandelowski, M. & Barroso J. (2003) Classifying the findings in qualitative studies. *Qualitative Health Research*, 13 (7), 905–923.

Sim, J. & Sharp, K. (1998) A critical appraisal of the role of triangulation in nursing research. *International Journal of Nursing Studies*, 35, 23–31.

Smaling, A. (2003) Inductive, analogical, and communicative generalization. *International Journal of Qualitative Methods*, 2 (1). Article 5. Retrieved 31 March 2007 from: http://www.ualberta.ca/~iiqm/backissues/2_1/html/smaling.html

Smith, J.K. (1993) *After the Demise of Empiricism: the Problem of Judging Social and Education Inquiry.* Norwood, NJ, Ablex.

Smith, J.K. & Deemer, D.K. (2000) The problem of criteria in the age of relativism. In: N.K. Denzin & Y.S. Lincoln (eds), *Handbook of Qualitative Research* (2nd edn, pp. 877–896). Thousand Oaks, Calif., Sage.

Thorne, S. (1997) Phenomenological positivism and other problematic trends in health science research. *Qualitative Health Research*, 7 (2), 287–293.

Thorne, S., Con, A., McGuiness, L., McPherson, G. & Harris, S.R. (2004) Health care communication issues in multiple sclerosis: an interpretive description. *Qualitative Health Research*, 14 (10), 5–22.

Whittemore, R., Chase, S. & Mandle, C.L. (2001) Validity in qualitative research. *Qualitative Health Research*, 11 (4), 522–537.

Chapter 10

DEVELOPMENTS IN QUALITATIVE RESEARCH

Introduction

During the past decade, there has been an increasing demand for scientific integrity in health-related research. Health care professions, including occupational therapy and physical therapy, are committed to developing new knowledge and seeking evidence to support clinical decision-making through scientific studies. 'Scientifically collected data allow us to look beyond our biases at the reality of patients, their lives, and their resources and at how they benefit from our intervention' (Rothstein, 1996). These aims can only be fulfilled, however, if the research undertaken is rigorous and ethical. In this chapter, we will discuss a number of developments that focus on ensuring the integrity and contribution of qualitative research to evidence-based and client-centered practice. The developments we have chosen to discuss in this chapter include an increased recognition of the responsibilities inherent in the participant–researcher relationship, finding the 'evidence' in qualitative findings through meta-synthesis and meta-analysis, the use of qualitative research in conjunction with other research methodologies in mixed methods approaches, and using the Internet and email as qualitative research tools. We will conclude this chapter, and the book, by briefly summarizing the key issues involved in planning and conducting qualitative research that we have discussed in previous chapters.

The participant–researcher relationship in qualitative research

In Chapter 3 we discussed the ethical issues related to ensuring that research participants are fully informed and give voluntary consent, and that their confidentiality and anonymity are protected at all phases of the research process. However, doing ethically responsible research requires that the researcher negotiates participation with those involved, establishes a relationship of trust with participants, and is sensitive to the shifting nature of the participation that has been agreed upon (Birch & Miller, 2002). It is the quality of the relationship between researcher and participant that can provide access to the in-depth, rich data characteristic of qualitative research. As such, it has been identified as a social relationship by feminist researchers, such as Oakley (1981) and Smith (1987) that embodies the notions of power, friendship, rapport and interpretation (Birch & Miller, 2002). Qualitative research is often framed as cooperative research founded on the principles of equality, transparency and democracy (Tee & Lathlean, 2004). However, cooperative inquiry raises concerns about how to make explicit the often taken-for-granted messiness inherent in the research relationship. Qualitative researchers 'exercise particular kinds of interpretive and representational power; they define areas of inquiry, set boundaries around their investigation, choose participants, interpret data and create text that will be viewed as authorized knowledge' (Cohn & Lyons, 2003, p. 41). It becomes particularly imperative to address these concerns when conducting research with participants who are potentially vulnerable, for example individuals with a history of mental health problems (Tee & Lathlean, 2004) or women who have experienced physical or sexual abuse (Schachter *et al.*, 1999). The concept of reflexivity, discussed in Chapter 5, needs to be expanded to include a reflection on the dynamics of power inherent in research and an account of the negotiations that take place during the research process.

Feminist researchers have also reframed the idea of the participant and researcher as autonomous individuals in the research process as represented in the ethics review process. They ask the researcher to engage in a dialogic relationship with participants, 'to build connected and transformative, participatory and empowering relationships with those studied' (Edwards & Mauthner, 2002, p. 26). This involves the concept of *reciprocity*, an effort to ensure a give and take communication involving a degree of self-disclosure on the part of the researcher in order to build a relationship of trust and mutual respect. Within this complex relationship between participant and researcher there may be multiple layers of expectations and meaning attributed by the participant to the experience and various motivations for offering to take part in the research and for ongoing participation (Peel *et al.*, 2006). However, 'how health research is understood, perceived, and accounted for by those who participate in it remains under-researched' (Peel *et al.*, 2006, p. 1347). There are a few exceptions, for example studies conducted by Barnitt (1999), Grinyer (2004) and Peel *et al.* (2006). Such investigations are congruent with the philosophy of qualitative research and client-centered practice, but there is clearly a need for more research. Qualitative research approaches have the potential to ensure a systematic analysis of participants' accounts of research participation. Such research would contribute important information about the reasons participants are involved, their expectations of the research process and findings, and how they define 'harm' and 'risk'.

Increasingly, it is being recognized that research that is relevant to health care clients' needs and priorities will make a more effective contribution to health care than other research (Department of Health, 2000). Decisions about research topics and methodologies have been primarily made by the professional and academic community and focused on treatment advancements and determining the efficacy and effectiveness of interventions. Thus, much research reflects the professional perspective and agenda and these decisions rarely include input from health care clients or consumer groups. Some advocacy consumer groups have consistently expressed their concerns that medical and health care research has served to exploit and oppress research participants, misrepresent the experience and reality of living with a disability or chronic illness, and further marginalize minority groups within society (Barnes & Mercer, 2004).

There is also an increasing awareness that the insights and perspectives of health care consumers are essential for the development of a client-centered and relevant research agenda, particularly in rehabilitation (Weaver *et al.*, 2001; Williamson, 2001). Participatory action research, which we discussed in Chapter 4, is concerned with producing knowledge that is directly useful to a group of people through cooperative action and the empowerment of people through the process of constructing and using their own knowledge (Reason, 1998). The interests of those involved in participatory action research have to be taken into account at every phase of the research. It is fundamentally committed to working towards positive change and ensuring that research findings are translated into real results. It is premised on the principles of democratic collaboration, respect and inclusivity and, as such, it is clearly consistent with the philosophy of client-centered practice and has much to contribute to health care research based on the different perspectives of clients and health care providers (Stringer & Genat, 2004). Other criticisms of health research focus on the failure of researchers 'to advocate for and work for change, apparently hoping instead that other people will read their research report and act on it' (Hammell, 2006, p. 175). A response to these criticisms has been a growing interest in developing ways by which qualitative research findings can be systematically incorporated into reviews. The rationale for this is that isolated qualitative studies do not in themselves contribute significantly to effective knowledge translation.

Qualitative meta-synthesis

The Cochrane Collaboration is an organization that aims to help people make well-informed decisions about health care by preparing, maintaining and promoting the accessibility of systematic reviews of the effects of health care interventions (Upshur, 2000). These systematic reviews have focused on the evidence derived from quantitative research and criteria for judging the quality of quantitative studies. A hierarchy of designs based on the strength of the evidence for treatment decisions has been established since the 1990s (Sackett *et al.*, 2000). The establishment of the Cochrane Qualitative Methods Group (2002) reflects a growing interest in understanding and evaluating the knowledge derived from qualitative research. This group has identified a number of ways that rigorous qualitative research can contribute to practice, policy and education, for example in understanding how an intervention is experienced by all those involved in developing, delivering and receiving interventions, what aspects of the intervention they value or not and why, or investigating professional, managerial or consumer behavior and external factors which facilitate or hinder successful implementation of a program or service. An increasing number of qualitative systematic reviews or meta-syntheses are being reported in the literature. The main barrier to determining the evidence derived from qualitative research, however, is that of developing clear criteria for selecting and appraising high-quality qualitative studies (see Chapter 9) for inclusion in reviews (Daly *et al.*, 2007).

Systematic review of relevant research literature and meta-analysis of research findings are central premises of evidence-based practice and conventional approaches to systematic review and meta-analysis have been primarily developed in relation to quantitative research. Qualitative studies have not as yet been 'optimally combined, contrasted, compared, and integrated with other qualitative work, thus failing to [provide evidence to] inform practice, create substantive and formal theory, and influence policy' (McCormick *et al.*, 2003, p. 933). This criticism draws attention to a number of fundamental philosophical and practical challenges in conducting qualitative research reviews related to the nature of the literature search strategies to be adopted (Barroso *et al.*, 2003), 'finding the findings in qualitative studies' (Sandelowski & Barroso, 2002, p. 213), and evaluating qualitative 'evidence' (Morse *et al.*, 2002), which we discussed in Chapter 9.

A systematic review involves identifying as many relevant studies as possible and critically appraising and comparing them to determine the quality of evidence that can be derived from them. Such a review, developed for quantitative research studies, traditionally proceeds through a series of well-defined and reproducible steps and may include statistical analysis of the aggregated data, usually of randomized controlled trials (CRTs), in order to detect a significant cause and effect relationship between a particular intervention and specific health outcomes (Campbell *et al.*, 2003). This statistical analysis is more accurately called meta-analysis, although the phrase is commonly used interchangeably with systematic review (Walsh & Downe, 2005).

A systematic review of qualitative studies follows similar steps to those conducted for quantitative research studies. These are: conducting a database and relevant literature search, deciding what to include, critically appraising potential studies, synthesizing and reporting the findings, and discussing the implications (Walsh & Downe, 2005). The term 'meta-synthesis' is generally used more commonly in the qualitative research literature than 'systematic review'. It is defined as:

> A complete study that involves rigorously examining and interpreting the findings (versus the raw data) of a number of qualitative research studies using qualitative methods. The goal of meta-synthesis is to produce a new and integrative interpretation of findings that is more substantive than those resulting from individual investigations (Finfgeld, 2003, p. 984).

In order to achieve this goal, a rigorous approach to synthesizing the findings needs to be adopted. The choice of analysis approach relates to the desired outcome of the meta-synthesis, that is, descriptive, theory explication or theory building. Where the goal is to provide a rich description of the topic of interest, a narrative or basic thematic analysis approach can be used, similar to that discussed earlier in Chapter 7. This type of descriptive synthesis summarizes or provides a description of the relevant research with minimal reinterpretation of the published data.

Where the analysis is directed toward creating themes of high explanatory value or developing theory, a constant comparison method generally associated with grounded theory, a meta-ethnographic approach or a content analysis approach is recommended. These approaches focus on an interpretive form of knowledge synthesis by generating a new interpretation from the cumulative published research findings. The aim is to produce a composite analysis to capture the essence or new dimensions of a phenomenon.

In the current absence of examples of meta-synthesis of qualitative studies in the physical therapy and occupational therapy literature, we have provided some informative nursing examples relevant to rehabilitation practice. Evans & FitzGerald (2002) conducted a systematic review (meta-synthesis) of the reasons for physically restraining patients and residents and provide detailed information about their process and their use of content analysis to synthesize the findings. Kearney (2001) conducted a meta-synthesis of fifteen qualitative papers focused on the topic of women's experience of domestic violence. She provides a detailed explanation of how she used a grounded theory approach to analyze the integrated findings. Thomas *et al.* (2004) demonstrated how the results of qualitative research and clinical randomized trials could be integrated, by conducting a systematic review. The review question was: 'What is known about the barriers to, and facilitators of, healthy eating among children aged 4–10 years?' (p. 1010). The authors assessed the quality of the studies that met the pre-specified inclusion criteria according to standards established for each methodological approach. They conducted a meta-analysis of the data from CRTs and a meta-synthesis of the qualitative study findings, and then combined them to answer the review question. This approach to systematic review allowed the integration of quantitative estimates of benefit and harm with qualitative understanding from people's lives and contributed to the development of more appropriate and effective interventions.

Meta-analysis is fundamentally different from meta-synthesis in that it depends on access to raw data. It involves analyzing the underlying assumptions of the data analysis process of each included study, comparing the different forms of data in terms of quality and contribution to the overall findings, and the synthesis of the findings as they relate to the phenomenon of interest. For example McCormick *et al.* (2003) conducted a qualitative meta-analysis of their own related studies to examine the context of health care and health care relationships.

Both approaches – meta-synthesis and meta-analysis – are discussed in depth in the nursing literature for those who wish to learn more, for example Finfgeld (2003) and Thorne *et al.* (2004). As discussed in Chapter 9, there is an increasing interest in developing more standardized approaches to classifying the findings of health qualitative studies and developing levels and applications of qualitative research evidence. Despite the increasing debate, approaches to qualitative research meta-synthesis and the classification of qualitative evidence are still at an early stage of development and there is as yet little consensus on the optimal approach. The task will be to reach a consensus about how studies are chosen for inclusion in meta-syntheses, how the quality of studies is assessed, what synthesis approach to use, and how the integrity of the synthesis findings can be established. However, qualitative meta-synthesis does appear to offer a promising approach to accumulating qualitative evidence and making it more accessible for clinicians and policy decision-makers.

Mixed methods

Interest in employing mixed methods strategies, particularly in health research, has been increasing (Morgan, 1998; Creswell, 2003). This growing interest in mixed methods research, as a means of systematically addressing the complexities of living with disability or chronic conditions, and of clinical practice and health service delivery, has further highlighted the need for occupational therapists and physical therapists to develop a critical understanding of both qualitative and quantitative approaches. As Morgan (1998) suggests, a program of studies that enable the health professional to alternate between qualitative and quantitative projects devoted to the same phenomenon would be ideal. Mixed method research is about forging an overall or negotiated account of the findings that brings together both components of the conversation or debate in order that the qualitative and quantitative findings can mutually inform the topic of interest (Bryman, 2007).

A mixed methods approach can be broadly defined as 'research in which the investigator collects and analyzes data, integrates the findings, and draws inferences using both qualitative and quantitative approaches or methods in a single study or a program of inquiry' (Tashakkori & Creswell, 2007). The central aim of such research is the integration of the two approaches. It is generally thought to be unreasonable that one person would have the necessary expertise to direct all aspects of a mixed methods study. The best way to support studies that combine qualitative and quantitative methods is to develop teams that can bring together specialists in both kinds of research design (Morgan, 1998; Bryman, 2007). However, this can create what Morgan (1998) calls 'isolated pools of knowledge' (p. 373), making it difficult to effectively integrate an objectivist methodology with a constructivist one based on people's discursive accounts (Bryman, 2007).

The decision to conduct mixed methods research begins, as with all types of research, with the formulation of the research question or purpose, and careful consideration by all involved in the research of the larger, theoretical perspective that will serve to guide the entire design, for example the social model of disability or critical theory. An explicitly articulated theoretical perspective can operate as a unifying and guiding framework regardless of the priority and implementation strategies subsequently chosen in designing the research (Creswell, 2003).

Having established a coherent purpose, the research design decision hinges on assigning priority to either the qualitative or quantitative approach and determining the sequencing of the methods. The priority decision focuses on the extent to which either the qualitative or quantitative method will be the principal approach to data collection and analysis. The real sequencing decision is how to connect different types of information to maximize their contributions to the success of the overall research project (Morgan, 1998). Creswell (2003) provides a detailed description of six sequencing designs: sequential explanatory, sequential exploratory, sequential transformative, concurrent triangulation, concurrent nested and concurrent transformative, and a useful discussion of their associated purposes. A mixed methods approach also requires a careful selection of sampling techniques. Teddlie & Yu (2007) introduce the concept of a probability-mixed-purposive sampling continuum and a number of useful mixed methods sampling strategies to assist researchers in making these decisions.

Research conducted to investigate strength training in young people with cerebral palsy (Dodd *et al.*, 2003; McBurney *et al.*, 2003; Taylor *et al.*, 2004) illustrates a mixed methods approach using a sequential explanatory design. According to Creswell (2003) this is 'the most straightforward of the six major mixed method approaches' and is usually 'characterized by the collection and analysis of quantitative data followed by collection and analysis of qualitative data' (p. 215). The initial study comprised a randomized controlled trial to evaluate the effects of strength training in young people with cerebral palsy. A qualitative exploration of the positive and negative outcomes of a home-based strength-training program (McBurney *et al.*, 2003) and factors that influence adherence to the program (Taylor *et al.*, 2004) was subsequently conducted. Young people with cerebral palsy (and their parents) who had completed a progressive resistance-training program were invited to participate in the qualitative study when they attended a follow-up measurement session held three months after. The authors suggested that the qualitative component made the following contributions: it provided additional evidence that strength training can be beneficial for young people with cerebral palsy, useful indicators to guide future quantitative studies of outcomes that are meaningful for people with cerebral palsy and clinically relevant information about factors that improved adherence to exercise programs. Mixed methods research employing a sequential design is rarely structured as one report. As with this example, researchers typically organize the report of procedures and findings into the quantitative and qualitative components, which are published separately, sometimes in different journals. In this situation, the authors can be expected to comment on how the qualitative findings elaborated or extended the quantitative results (Creswell, 2003). In other mixed methods designs, for example in a concurrent design where the aim is not to distinguish the quantitative and qualitative phase, the data collection methods would be described separately but the findings would be combined and integrated (Creswell, 2003).

Concerns have been raised in the past that some mixed methods designs treat the qualitative research component as tentative until "confirmed" by the quantitative research component. Morgan (1998) argues that this is largely a matter of perception but Morse & Richards (2002) caution that ensuring 'methodological integrity' is especially relevant when researchers combine ontological and epistemological positions in conducting mixed methods research. The contribution of mixed methods research to evidence-based practice in health care depends on the degree to which mixed methods researchers genuinely integrate their findings (Bryman, 2007). Bryman (2007) identified a number of barriers encountered by researchers attempting to construct a negotiated account of their findings. These are related to the practicalities of conducting research, for example timelines and sequencing of research projects, compartmentalization of researcher skills and theoretical perspectives, and the relative absence of 'exemplars' of mixed methods research in the literature. The latter concern is particularly pertinent for occupational therapists and physical therapists. However, there are a growing number of resources dedicated to the discussion and dissemination of mixed methods research that are available to those who are interested in these approaches, in the form of books, for example Tashakkori & Teddlie (2003) and Creswell (2003), and journals, for example the *Journal of Mixed Methods Research*.

Internet recruitment and email interviews

The rapid development of the World Wide Web and access by large numbers of people to email has made it possible for qualitative researchers to recruit participants through the Internet and conduct interviews via email. These developments have the potential to overcome some of the barriers encountered in conventional research approaches but they also raise methodological and ethical issues that have not as yet been systematically debated in the literature (Mann & Stewart, 2000). Illingworth (2001) warns of the need 'to avoid use of the Internet as an "easy option" and [to] encourage a more developed focus on the justification, applicability and benefits of Internet research to particular projects' (para. 1.1). As with any research approach, the effective use of computer mediated communication is dependent on what is being researched, who is being researched and why. Most sampling strategies in qualitative research are concerned primarily with the participants' ability to reflect on the complexity of a specific phenomenon and contribute to a rich description of it. Internet sampling is similarly driven by the research question and the need to access those with experience and knowledge of the topic of interest. Practically, the researcher needs to select the most appropriate Internet site and seek permission from the site moderator to place an announcement of the study to optimize the chance of recruiting individuals interested in the specific topic (Illingworth, 2001). Examples of such sites might be professional organizations that are accessed by members, or advocacy organizations providing support and information for the general public. Advantages of this recruitment strategy are that it is not necessary to collaborate with clinical sites or involve gatekeepers, it is easy to achieve geographical diversity and, potentially, there is easier access to disabled people (Hamilton & Bowers, 2006). In addition, this recruitment strategy fulfills the ethics review requirements that the participants initiate their involvement in a study, thus ensuring that it is voluntary and that they can withdraw at any time. The disadvantages relate to the possibility of participant fraud, that is, anyone may pose as a research participant, and reliance on the Internet precludes representation of those who do not have, or have limited, access to the Internet (Illingworth, 2001). Hamilton & Bowers (2006) suggest that in addressing the 'data fraud' issue, 'researchers might have to depend on other screening methods' (p. 824), such as sending hard copy consent forms to participants' home addresses, requesting official identification for compensation purposes and making phone calls to confirm study information. There are real concerns that conducting research through Internet and email access simply 'reinforces existing social divisions between the "information rich" – those who have access to computers and online facilities – and the "information poor" – those who do not' (Illingworth, 2001, para. 12.1). However, these issues may be more or less problematic depending on the nature and purpose of the proposed study. Let us consider a hypothetical study exploring the experiences of physical therapists and occupational therapists working for non-governmental organizations in developing countries. As part of the participant recruitment strategy, the researcher could seek permission to solicit volunteers on a variety of professional association web sites. Participants accessed in this way would have access to the resources needed and their identity would be verifiable. Since they would be located around the world, an email interview would be a plausible choice of data collection method.

As we have discussed in Chapter 6, focused interview or in-depth interview is the most common data collection method used in qualitative research. Email interviews can be more convenient for both participant and researcher in that arrangements are greatly simplified and email interview contributions can be made at any time during a specified period of time. According to Hamilton & Bowers (2006) although the researcher can maintain the topic focus during the email interview it does enable the participant a measure of control of the research process not so evident in the more conventional interview situation. Owing to the asynchronous nature of email interviews, both the researcher and participants have time to reflect on the questions and their responses. For the researcher, email interviewing also facilitates ongoing analysis. Researchers have time to analyze the participants' responses and develop more clarifying questions or ask for more details. 'If more than one interview is taking place in the same time frame, comparison across interviews can occur' (Hamilton & Bowers, 2006, p. 831) and negative cases can be explored. As discussed in Chapter 3, the data acquired through audio or videotaping the face-to-face interview need to be transcribed in order to convert it to written form. In email interviewing, transcription is not necessary and this may be viewed as an advantage in that it eliminates the need for taping equipment and the issues of reliability, confidentiality and expense associated with getting the data transcribed. The availability of an audit or decision trail, discussed in Chapter 9, can contribute to the trustworthiness of the research. Establishing an audit trail would be easier in email interviewing as all communication between researcher and participant could be printed and hard copies stored.

Email interviewing is not comparable to the personal interaction that is characteristic of face-to-face interviewing. There are legitimate concerns that the nuances involved in face-to-face verbal communication are lost, and 'the lack of physicality and reliance on written information potentially leads to the loss of important observational elements and cues vital to the validation of the researcher–participant interaction' (Illingworth, 2001, para. 14.3). Mann & Stewart (2000) counter these concerns by saying that the loss of visual cues might not be of central importance as, in reality, interpretations of body language or other physical cues are rarely incorporated as data. However, we consider that their opinion is controversial and that many qualitative researchers would place a greater value on the quality of the relationship and contextual understanding that can be achieved in a face-to-face interview. It is clear that email interviewers need to develop a different set of skills in order to establish trust and rapport between individuals linked only by a computer interface (Illingworth, 2001). These skills would include, aside from computer and typing abilities, the ability to moderate, communicate effectively and redirect the dialogue using a keyboard. It is possible that in some circumstances respondents would welcome and be encouraged by the anonymity and privacy inherent in email interviewing.

There are also concerns that email communication tends to be superficial or practical in nature and perhaps not suited for the sort of in-depth, thoughtful and reflective communication that is the goal of qualitative research. Advocates for this method counter by saying that email interviews, like face-to-face, are embedded in the philosophical approach that supports the research design, and that 'this changes the nature of the communication regardless of the data collection method' (Hamilton & Bowers, 2006, p. 829). Increasingly, people are adept at using email as a communication tool and can effectively share their experiences and opinions with clarity and conviction (Mann & Stewart, 2000). Hamilton & Bowers (2006) recommend explaining to potential participants that their contributions to an email interview are more like 'answering an essay question, so that they are not under the impression that they would be providing simple yes or no answers' (p. 830).

The ethical issues of informed consent and confidentiality are similar to those associated with traditional interviews and involve establishing password controlled computer files, locked storage for hard copies of communication, use of participant pseudonyms or codes, permission to seek additional information about the study from someone other than the researcher and the facility to withdraw at any time. Hamilton & Bowers (2006) recommend providing the participant with a hard copy of the informed consent form for signing, as a tangible representation of the study and as a means of guarding against data fraud. Internet participant recruitment and email interviewing as a data collection method offer new alternatives to be considered in designing a qualitative study. However, identifying the research question or purpose remains central to guiding the ensuing research design and the decision to use Internet participant recruitment and email interviewing, as with any sampling and method choices, needs to be rigorously justified.

Conclusion

Our purpose in writing this book was to provide occupational therapists and physical therapists interested in learning more about qualitative research with as comprehensive and practical a resource as possible. Qualitative research has typically been discussed by comparing and contrasting it with the assumptions, techniques and strategies developed for quantitative research. In this book, while a certain amount of comparison is unavoidable, we wanted to focus on the different approaches to qualitative research and their contribution to generating knowledge in rehabilitation. Our discussions have been premised on our conviction that the research endeavor is not an atheoretical or dispassionate one. As researchers, we enter the research process with established theoretical orientations, professional and personal knowledge and experience. These may be explicit or taken for granted, but in either case they exert considerable influence on how we read and interpret the research literature, on the research questions we ask, and the studies we design. In Chapter 1, we made the argument that all research is interpretive and not a neutral or objective undertaking. It is essential in conducting qualitative research to make our theoretical orientations transparent, and to assist readers to achieve this objective we discussed the contexts of professional practice and rehabilitation and several models of disability and rehabilitation. In qualitative research, the researcher's theoretical orientation, experience and background knowledge contribute to the conceptual framework that bounds and focuses the evolving research proposal. As Miles & Huberman (1994) suggest, 'conceptual frameworks are simply the current version of the researcher's knowledge of the terrain being investigated. As the explorer's knowledge of the terrain deepens, the map becomes correspondingly more differentiated and integrated' (p. 20).

In Chapter 2, we examined the key philosophical systems of interpretivism, constructivism and critical theory that underpin the unique characteristics of qualitative research and the types of professional knowledge and reasoning congruent with qualitative research. We also discussed evidence-based practice and client-centered practice as two of the most influential concepts in rehabilitation although, as Hammell (2006) suggests, 'these terms are rarely used by the same authors' (p. 177). The two practice approaches have been portrayed in the past as incompatible. It is now generally acknowledged, however, that evidence-based practice depends upon 'the integration of best research evidence with clinical expertise and patient values' (Sackett *et al.*, 2000, p. 1). This broader definition of evidence-based practice is more applicable to the multi-factorial nature of rehabilitation practice and highlights the urgent need to incorporate the client's values, priorities, experience and knowledge into decision-making at all levels of health care. The characteristics of qualitative research are congruent with the underlying philosophy of client-centered practice and, as such, it has an increasingly important role to play in bringing these two important concepts together for the benefit of rehabilitation clients.

Elements of both practice approaches are represented in an organizing framework for decision-making in rehabilitation, devised by Pollock & Rochon (2002) to support practice decisions. The E Model, as it is called, consists of five categories that represent the complexity of rehabilitation practice: expectations, environment, experience, ethics and evidence. Qualitative research has the potential to contribute to our understanding in all five categories. The category of expectations addresses one of the central tenets of client-centered practice, that the client identifies and articulates the goals and expectations upon which the therapy process is based. The environmental factors that influence the nature of therapeutic practice can take many forms and exist at the macro-level, for example health care policy and resource allocation, at the institutional or community meso-level, and at the micro-level of the therapeutic relationship and interaction between the client and practitioner. Environmental factors include cultural and societal norms and values that will also influence the decisions made and services offered.

The therapists' experience 'is a powerful force influencing decision-making' (Pollock & Rochon, 2002, p. 35). It encompasses the formal learning gained from professional education and continuing education, and the more informal learning that occurs from the development of new ideas in practice, reflection on current knowledge, and the application and synthesis of that evolving knowledge into practice (Higgs & Titchen, 2001). The role of ethics has increasingly become an important topic of discussion in health care, particularly in rehabilitation settings, where the ethical issues are different from acute care and more representative of the complex, holistic and multidisciplinary context of rehabilitation. As Pollock & Rochon (2002) point out, 'clinical reasoning is not situationally specific; it draws on the values, beliefs, philosophies and culture of the [practitioner]' (p. 37). The fifth category in the E Model – the use of "best" evidence – has perhaps had the greatest influence on clinical reasoning in recent years. Traditionally, as we have discussed, the concept of evidence was associated with quantitative research, but there is an increasing recognition of the contribution qualitative research evidence can make to our understanding of the complexity of rehabilitation and the decisions to be made with clients living with disability and chronic conditions.

Research questions arise from foreshadowed problems and clinical irritants experienced by occupational therapists and physical therapists in practice. Qualitative research is ideal for addressing questions that begin with *how* or *what* and that direct us to describe or explore phenomena of which little is known. In Chapter 3, we provided an overview of the research design process and practical tips on how to plan and execute a qualitative study. The question not only informs the type of research but also the choice of methodology, methods of data collection and data analysis approach. We have argued that the application of an appropriate methodology – phenomenology, grounded theory, ethnography and participatory action research – contributes to a coherent research design. A range of data collection methods – in-depth interviews, focus groups, participant observation, consensus techniques and unobtrusive methods – are associated with qualitative research and were discussed in Chapter 5. The choice of method needs to be congruent with the nature of the research question and the guiding methodology; for example, a phenomenological study that explores the perspectives of the individual would primarily use in-depth interviewing. Data collection can only occur after participants have volunteered to be involved in the study. The sampling strategies associated with qualitative research clearly illustrate the differences between qualitative and quantitative approaches. The aim of sampling in qualitative research is to deliberately select and recruit people who have experience, knowledge or expertise of a particular phenomenon or situation. Participant involvement in qualitative research is much more than the concept of sampling or selection implies. The quality of qualitative research, in large part, depends on the relationship of trust and rapport that the researcher can develop with the participants, and many of the ethical issues characteristic of qualitative research emanate from this central relationship. Qualitative data usually take a text-based or narrative form and novice researchers are occasionally surprised at the quantity of data that can be generated from a relatively uncomplicated study. Efficient management of the data is an important skill that we discussed in Chapter 6. The data analysis process is often the least well described and justified aspect of a qualitative research report. In Chapter 7, we described a basic thematic approach to qualitative data analysis. This type of approach is foundational to the more detailed and specialized approaches associated with specific methodologies, such as grounded theory. The contribution of qualitative research to generating new knowledge and its applicability to practice depends, as with any type of research, on establishing the rigor and quality of the design and findings. Criteria by which a qualitative study can be critically appraised, and strategies to enhance the design and confirm the findings, have been developed (see Chapter 9), but these continue to be the focus of much debate in the qualitative literature. The elements of qualitative research design that we have introduced in this book are summarized in Table 10.1.

In order for qualitative research to make a significant contribution to knowledge transfer and the generation of evidence to support clinical reasoning, the findings must be disseminated through presentation and publication. In Chapter 8, we made the case that it is the researcher's responsibility to ensure that subsequent articles and professional presentations accurately represent the participant's perspectives, are accessible for them to read and will benefit them. We concluded this book with a discussion of interesting new developments in qualitative research that will challenge and fascinate those of us committed to conducting and promoting qualitative research in occupational therapy and physical therapy in the future. We consider it important that our professions be knowledgeable of both the qualitative and quantitative paradigms. We were motivated to write this book by our enthusiasm and commitment to qualitative research and we hope that it will prove useful to those occupational therapists and physical therapists interested in critically appraising and conducting qualitative research.

Table 10.1 Overview of qualitative research approaches.

| Characteristics | Interpretivism | Theoretical traditions | | Critical theory |
| | | Constructivism Methodologies | | |
	Phenomenology descriptive or hermeneutic (interpretive)	Grounded theory	Ethnography	Participatory action research (PAR)
Central aim of research	Search for individual central underlying meaning (essence) of an experience or phenomenon	Systematic analytic approach to the generation or discovery of a substantive theory	Develop a rich description that facilitates a greater understanding of the experiences of people within a cultural group	Systematic production of knowledge and action directly useful to a group of people – through research, adult education, and sociopolitical action – and empowerment of group members through the process
Main methods	In-depth interviews (small number)	In-depth interviews (large number) Non-obtrusive methods	Participant observation In-depth interviews Focus groups Non-obtrusive methods	Any (both narrative and numerical) depending on research phase
Participant recruitment	Purposive sampling	Initial purposive sampling Theoretical sampling Discriminant sampling	Purposive sampling Key informants Gatekeepers	Purposive sampling Dynamic roles

Associated concepts	Essence Bracketing (époche)	Data saturation Theoretical sensitivity Sensitizing concepts Theory verification	'Thick' description Insider (emic) Outsider (etic) Fieldwork Immersion	Stakeholders Underlying principles of democratic action, participation, empowerment, and respect Cyclical model of research (planning, acting, observing and reflecting)
Data analysis process	Thematic analysis Interpretive phenomenological analysis (Smith, 2003), Colaizzi's (1978) method	Constant comparison method Coding (open, line-by-line, axial, selective) Dimensionalization Conditional matrix	Iterative process Thematic analysis Search for inconsistencies and contradictions	Data analysis relates to data collection method
Associated strategies of rigor	Member checking Reflexivity Audit trail	Analytic memos Reflexivity Data triangulation	Member checking Prolonged engagement Data saturation	Based on a series of achievable objectives Detailed record of developmental and continuous cyclical process
Prominent authors (see Chapter 4 reference list)	Giorgi (1997) Giorgi & Giorgi (2003a) Moustakas (1994) van Manen (1990)	Glaser & Strauss (1967) Glaser (1992) Strauss & Corbin (1990; 1994) Charmaz (2000)	Hammersley & Atkinson (1995) Spradley (1979)	Reason (1998) Reason & Bradbury (2001)

References

Barnes, C. & Mercer, G. (2004) Theorising and researching disability from a social model perspective. In: C. Barnes & G. Mercer (eds), *Implementing the Social Model of Disability: the Theory and Research* (pp. 1–17). Leeds, The Disability Press.

Barnitt, R. & Partridge, C. (1999) The legacy of being a research subject: follow-up studies of participants in therapy research. *Physiotherapy Research International*, 4 (4), 250–261.

Barroso, J., Gollop, C.J., Sandelowski, M., Meynell, J., Pearce, P.F. & Collins, L. (2003) The challenges of searching and retrieving qualitative studies. *Western Journal of Nursing Research*, 25 (2), 153–178.

Birch, M. & Miller, T. (2002) Encouraging participation: ethics and responsibilities. In: M. Mauthner, M. Birch, J. Jessop & T. Miller (eds), *Ethics in Qualitative Research* (pp. 91–106). London, Sage.

Bryman, A. (2007) Barriers to integrating quantitative and qualitative research. *Journal of Mixed Methods Research*, 1 (1), 8–22.

Campbell, R., Pound, P., Pope, C. *et al.* (2003) Evaluating meta-ethnography: a synthesis of qualitative research on lay experiences of diabetes and diabetes care. *Social Science & Medicine*, 56, 671–684.

Cochrane Qualitative Methods Group (2002) Retrieved 12 March 2007 from: http://www.joannabriggs.edu.au/cqrmg/index.html

Cohn, E. & Lyons, K.D. (2003) The perils of power in interpretive research. *American Journal of Occupational Therapy*, 57 (1), 40–48.

Colaizzi, P.F. (1978) Psychological research as the phenomenologist views it. In: R.S. Valle & M. King (eds), *Existential Phenomenological Alternatives for Psychology* (pp. 48–71). New York, Oxford University Press.

Creswell, J.W. (2003) *Research Design, Qualitative, Quantitative, and Mixed Approaches* (2nd edn, pp. 208–225). Thousand Oaks, Calif., Sage.

Department of Health (2000) *The Expert Patient: a New Approach to Chronic Disease Management for the Twenty-first Century.* London, Department of Health.

Dodd, K.J., Taylor, N.F. & Graham, H.K. (2003) A randomized clinical trial of strength training in young people with cerebral palsy. *Developmental Medicine and Child Neurology*, 45, 652–657.

Edwards, R. & Mauthner, M. (2002) Ethics and feminist research: theory and practice. In: M. Mauthner, M. Birch, J. Jessop & T. Miller (eds), *Ethics in Qualitative Research* (pp. 14–31). London, Sage.

Evans, D. & FitzGerald, M. (2002) Reasons for physically restraining patients and residents: a systematic review and content analysis. *International Journal of Nursing Studies*, 39, 735–743.

Finfgeld, D.L. (2003) Meta-synthesis: the state of the art – so far. *Qualitative Health Research*, 13 (7), 893–904.

Grinyer, A. (2004) The narrative correspondence method: what a follow-up study can tell us about the longer term effect on participants in emotionally demanding research. *Qualitative Health Research*, 14, 1326–1341.

Hamilton, R.J. & Bowers, B.J. (2006) Internet recruitment and email interviews in qualitative studies. *Qualitative Health Research*, 16 (6), 821–835.

Hammell, K.W. (2006) *Perspectives on Disability & Rehabilitation: Contesting Assumptions, Challenging Practice.* Edinburgh, Churchill Livingstone Elsevier.

Higgs, J. & Titchen, A. (2001) *Practice Knowledge & Expertise in the Health Professions.* Oxford, Butterworth Heinemann.

Illingworth, N. (2001) The Internet matters: exploring the use of the Internet as a research tool. *Sociological Research Online*, 6 (2). Retrieved 22 March 2007 from: http://www.socresonline.org.uk/6/2/illingworth.html

Kearney, M.H. (2001) Enduring love: a grounded formal theory of women's experience of domestic violence. *Research in Nursing & Health*, 24, 270–282.

Mann, C. & Stewart, F. (2000) *Internet Communication and Qualitative Research: a Handbook for Researching Online*. London, Sage.

McBurney, H., Taylor, N.F., Dodd, K.J. & Graham, H.K. (2003) A qualitative analysis of the benefits of strength training for young people with cerebral palsy. *Developmental Medicine and Child Neurology*, 45, 658–663.

McCormick, J., Rodney, P. & Varcoe, C. (2003) Reinterpretations across studies: an approach to meta-analysis. *Qualitative Health Research*, 13 (7), 933–944.

Miles, M.B. & Huberman, A.M. (1994) *Qualitative Data Analysis* (2nd edn). Thousand Oaks, Calif., Sage.

Morgan, D. (1998) Practical strategies for combining qualitative and quantitative methods: applications to health research. *Qualitative Health Research*, 8 (3), 362–376.

Morse, J.M. & Richards, L. (2002) *Read Me First for a User's Guide to Qualitative Methods*. Thousand Oaks, Calif., Sage.

Morse, J., Barrett, M., Kayan, M., Olson, K. & Spiers, J. (2002) Verification strategies for establishing reliability and validity in qualitative research. *International Journal of Qualitative Methods*, 1 (2), 1–19.

Oakley, A. (1981) Interviewing women: a contradiction in terms. In: H. Roberts (ed.), *Doing Feminist Research* (pp. 30–61). London, Routledge.

Peel, E., Parry, O., Douglas, M. & Lawton, J. (2006) 'It's no skin off my nose': why people participate in qualitative research. *Qualitative Health Research*, 16 (10), 1335–1349.

Pollock, N. & Rochon, S. (2002) Becoming an evidence-based practitioner. In: M. Law (ed.), *Evidence-based Rehabilitation: a Guide to Practice* (pp. 31–46). Thorofare, NJ, Slack.

Reason, P. (1998) Three approaches to participative inquiry. In: N.K. Denzin & Y.S. Lincoln (eds), *Strategies of Qualitative Inquiry* (pp. 261–291). Thousand Oaks, Calif., Sage.

Reason, P. & Bradbury, H. (eds) (2001) *Handbook of Action Research: Participative Inquiry and Practice*. London, Sage.

Rothstein, J.M. (1996) Editor's note: outcome and survival. *Physical Therapy*, 76 (2), 126.

Sackett, D.L., Straus, S.E., Richardson, W.S., Rosenburg, W. & Haynes, R.B. (2000) *Evidence-based Medicine: How to Practice and Teach EBM* (2nd edn). Edinburgh, Churchill Livingstone.

Sandelowski, M. & Barroso, J. (2002) Finding the findings in qualitative studies. *Journal of Nursing Scholarship*, 34 (3), 213–219.

Schachter, C., Stalker, C. & Teram, E. (1999) Toward sensitive practice: issues for physical therapists working with survivors of childhood abuse. *Physical Therapy*, 79 (3), 248–261.

Smith, D. (1987) *The Everyday World as Problematic: a Feminist Sociology*. Toronto, Ont., University of Toronto.

Smith, J.A. (2003) *Qualitative Psychology: a Practical Guide to Research Methods*. London, Sage.

Stringer, E. & Genat, W.J. (2004) *Action Research in Health*. Upper Saddle River, NJ, Merrill Prentice Hall.

Tashakkori, A. & Creswell, J. (2007) Editorial: the new era of mixed methods. *Journal of Mixed Methods Research*, 1 (1), 3–7.

Tashakkori, A. & Teddlie, C. (eds) (2003) *Handbook of Mixed Methods in the Social and Behavior Sciences.* Thousand Oaks, Calif., Sage.

Taylor, N.F., Dodd, K.J., McBurney, H. & Graham, H.K. (2004) Factors influencing adherence to a home-based strength-training programme for young people with cerebral palsy. *Physiotherapy*, *90*, 57–63.

Teddlie, C. & Yu, F. (2007) Mixed method sampling: a typology with examples. *Journal of Mixed Methods Research*, *1* (1), 77–100.

Tee, S.R. & Lathlean, J.A. (2004) The ethics of conducting a cooperative inquiry with vulnerable people. *Journal of Advanced Nursing*, *47* (5), 536–543.

Thomas, J., Harden, A., Oakley, A. *et al.* (2004) Integrating qualitative research with trials in systematic reviews. *British Medical Journal*, *328* (24 April), 1010–1012.

Thorne, S., Jensen, L., Kearney, M.H., Noblit, G. & Sandelowski, M. (2004) Qualitative meta-synthesis: reflections on methodological orientation and ideological agenda. *Qualitative Health Research*, *14* (10), 1342–1365.

Upshur, R.E.G. (2000) The status of qualitative research as evidence. In: J.M. Morse, J.M. Swanson & A.J. Kuzel (eds), *The Nature of Qualitative Evidence* (pp. 5–26). Thousand Oaks, Calif., Sage.

Walsh, D. & Downe, S. (2005) Meta-synthesis method for qualitative research: a literature review. *Journal of Advanced Nursing*, *50* (2), 204–211.

Weaver, F., Guihan, M., Pape, T. *et al.* (2001) Creating a research agenda in SCI based on provider and consumer input. *SCI Psychosocial Process*, *14* (2), 77–88.

Williamson, C. (2001) Editorial: what does involving consumers in research mean? *Qualitative Journal of Medicine*, *94*, 661–664.

INDEX

New for 2007 and Online submission using Manuscript Central

PUBLISHED QUARTERLY

Learning in Health and Social Care

Editor: Pam Shakespeare

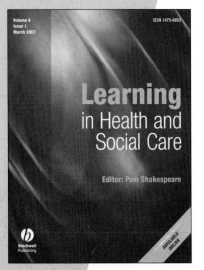

Volume 6
Issue 1
March 2007

ISSN 1473-6853

Learning
in Health and
Social Care

Editor: Pam Shakespeare

Blackwell
Publishing

AVAILABLE ONLINE

Learning in Health and Social Care is an international peer-reviewed journal contributing to the growth and development of knowledge about approaches to the facilitation of individual, team and organisational learning in a variety of professional environments. The journal publishes quality research on formal and non-formal learning for, in or through professional practice. As the journal addresses shared and common issues for the professions it appeals to many in the health and welfare sectors, including those interested in developing collaborative working and multiprofessional approaches to service delivery.

The journal accepts original papers and the results of literature reviews and commissioned studies. An Open Forum encourages the exchange of ideas, commentary and critical discourse, including reviews of relevant books. Articles that reflect collaborative working between and within professions are particularly welcome, as are research studies situated in one or more professions that raise issues relevant to several professions.

- **Promotes educational effectiveness**
- **Provides research-based evidence on key learning issues**
- **Explores multiprofessional learning in a variety of contexts**
- **Debates formal and informal learning in a range of settings**
- **Examines formal organisational learning, power, political relationships and resource challenges**
- **Delivers the latest policies and directives from statutory bodies for all the professions**

Manuscripts for submissions should be sent to the Editorial Assistant at:
LHSoffice@oxon.blackwellpublishing.com

Indexed/Abstracted in E-psyche; CareData; Contents Pages in Education; Educational Research in Abstracts

For more information, or to subscribe, please visit

www.blackwellpublishing.com/lhs

From here you can view online content in *Blackwell Synergy* and sign up for FREE e-mailed table of contents alerts.

Register FREE at *Blackwell Synergy* and

- Receive tables of contents email alerts directly to your desktop with links to article abstracts
- Search across all full text articles for key words or phrases
- Access free sample issues from every online journal
- Browse table of contents and abstracts for all journals, and save favourites on your own custom page

Published quarterly, ISSN 1473-6853